THE GUIDE TO
THE FUTURE OF MEDICINE

Technology AND The Human Touch

Bertalan Meskó

Publisher: Webicina Kft.
The Guide to the Future of Medicine: Technology AND the Human Touch
Bertalan Mesko

Copyright © 2014 by Dr. Bertalan Mesko
All rights reserved.

Editor: Dr. Richard E. Cytowic
Cover Design: Szilvia Kora
Interior Design: Roland Rekeczki

This book was self–published by the author under Webicina Kft. No part of this book may be reproduced in any form by any means without the express permission of the author. This includes reprints, excerpts, photocopying, recording, or any future means of reproducing text.

If you would like to do any of the above or need information on bulk purchases, please contact the author at http://medicalfuturist.com.

ISBN 978-963-12-0007-2

Printed by CreateSpace, An Amazon.com Company.
Printed in the United States of America.

References and illustration sources are provided.

The content of this book is for informational purposes only and does not constitute professional medical advice, legal advice, diagnosis, treatment or recommendation of any specific treatment or provider of any kind. Individuals should always seek the advice of qualified professionals with any questions or concerns about their health or treatment. Neither the author nor any of the content in this book is meant to recommend or endorse specific hospitals, physicians, cities, hotels, facilities, or procedures. We advise readers to do their own research and due diligence, make their own informed decisions and seek their own medical and legal advice. Reliance on any information provided in this book is solely at your own risk.

Table of contents

About the Author	vi
Foreword by Lucien Engelen	vii
Preface	ix
Part I. Introduction	1
Let's prepare for what is coming next	2
The role of a medical futurist	4
Part II. Trends That Are Shaping the Future of Medicine	5
The anatomy of a trend description	5
Trend 1. Empowered Patients	6
New online communities	9
E–patients are the hackers of healthcare	11
Trend 2. Gamifying Health	14
Persuading people to follow therapy	15
Video games and platforms in the hospital	18
Sticking to a therapy is hard	19
Trend 3. Eating in the future	21
Stem cell burgers and the world's healthiest food	22
Do you know what you eat?	24
Trend 4. Augmented Reality and Virtual Reality	29
From glass to contact lens and beyond	33
Trend 5. Telemedicine and Remote Care	37
House calls of the 21st century	39
Trend 6. Re–thinking the Medical Curriculum	43
How to design a new curriculum	47
Trend 7. Surgical and Humanoid Robots	50
Obstacles for wider adoption	52
Understanding the value of robotics	56
Robots among us	57
Trend 8. Genomics and Truly Personalized Medicine	61
Genome data for everyone	63
Genomics can change lives	65

Table of Contents

Trend 9. Body Sensors Inside and Out — 70
    Wearing invisible sensors — 71
    Constantly monitoring our health? — 77

Trend 10. The Medical Tricorder and Portable Diagnostics — 80
    Clinical laboratory and radiology at home — 82
    Evidence–based and customized Mobile Health — 83

Trend 11. Growing Organs in a Dish — 87
    The world of stem cells — 92

Trend 12. Do–It–Yourself Biotechnology — 95
    Biotechnology labs in the community — 98
    Biotech startups revolutionizing medicine — 100

Trend 13. The 3D Printing Revolution — 102
    3D printing to go mainstream — 103
    3D printing everything — 106

Trend 14. Iron Man: Powered exoskeletons and prosthetics — 111
    Customizing prosthetics — 116
    Neuroprosthetics — 119
    The ethical dilemmas — 120

Trend 15. The End of Human Experimentation — 122
    Simulating organs on chips — 125

Trend 16. Medical Decisions via Artificial Intelligence — 129
    The cost beyond — 132
    The friendly or unfriendly AI — 134

Trend 17. Nanorobots Living In Our Blood — 137
    Endless opportunities — 139
    Forming a new community — 141

Trend 18. Hospitals of the Future — 143
    Lessons for designing future hospitals — 145

Trend 19. Virtual–Digital Brains — 149
    Measuring EEG at home — 150
    Controlling neurons with optogenetics — 155
    Brain implants and neuroenhancement — 157
    Connecting brains and computers — 158

Table of Contents

Trend 20. The Rise of Recreational Cyborgs — 161
    The first cyborg ever — 164
    The Most Connected Man — 166
    Augmenting human capabilities — 169

Trend 21. Cryonics and Longevity — 171
    How long can we live? — 172

Trend 22. What Will a Brand New Society Look Like? — 175
    Technosexuality and beyond — 177

Part III: Preparing For the Future of Medicine — 181
    Keep yourself up-to-date — 181
    Embrace digital — 181
    Read, listen and watch — 181
    Look outside of medicine — 182
    Avoid hype — 182
    Extrapolate from today's trends — 182
    Forget about the ultimate solution — 182
    Don't get scared by the growing importance of technology — 183
    Don't overestimate technology — 183
    Don't give up if you lack IT skills — 183
    Fight to keep the human touch — 184
    Accept mutual relationships — 184
    Prepare others for the changes — 184
    Predicting the future of medicine is challenging — 184
    Communicate and crowdsource — 185

Conclusion — 186
Acknowledgements — 188
Illustration Sources — 189
References — 191

About the Author

Bertalan Mesko, MD, PhD is a medical futurist who graduated from the University of Debrecen Medical School and Health Science Center. He received the Weszprémy Award as a medical doctor and finished his PhD summa cum laude in the field of clinical genomics.

As a medical futurist, he envisions the next steps to be taken and the trends happening now in order to have a mutually positive relationship between the human touch and the innovative technologies that await us in the future of healthcare.

Dr. Mesko is the managing director and founder of Webicina.com, the first service that curates medical and health-related social media resources for patients and medical professionals. He has given over 500 presentations at institutions ranging from Yale, Stanford, and Harvard to the World Health Organization and the Futuremed course organized by the Singularity University. He is also a consultant for pharma and medical technology companies.

He is the author of the Social Media in Clinical Practice handbook, as well as the multiple award-winning medical blog, Scienceroll.com. He is the founder of and lecturer at the Social Media in Medicine online-and-offline university course, which is the first of its kind worldwide.

Dr. Mesko's work has been cited by CNN, the World Health Organization, Nature Medicine, The New York Times, Al Jazeera, the British Medical Journal, and Wired Science, among others.

He is a member of the World Future Society.

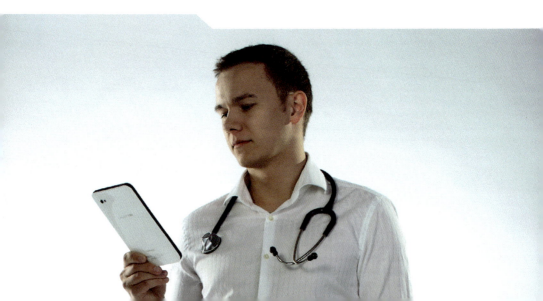

Foreword by Lucien Engelen

In fifty years from now, I expect more than 50% of the revenue in healthcare will come from companies that do not exist, or do not have any business in healthcare today.

Technological developments as well as changes in society will create the 5th democratization. After music, travel, retail and media; healthcare is next to be disrupted. Adding to that, the increasing patient empowerment brings in "the perfect storm" for health(care). In my keynotes I often use the 4D anagram: Delocalization, Digitalization, Dollars and Democratization. Because they are all tied together and starting to peak at somewhat the same time, it creates the ideal eco–system for autonomous change.

Change that will hit health(care) for a lot of people ‚overnight', not that this wasn't foreseeable, but the signs have been neglected over and over again. Medicine is starting to adopt new treatments, medications and protocols but is lacking far behind where it goes on reflecting on the model of health(care). We basically deliver healthcare the same way it was done a hundred years ago. Now due to the exponentially growing possibilities technology is bringing to the table, we, for instance, will start bringing back health(care) into the homes of people. This also brings the need of new payment models, changes in curriculum for medical students like the one that we've crafted at Radboud University Medical Center, or even new legislation.

For these kinds of transformational processes, we need people who can address these changes and paint a picture of the world of tomorrow. In my work of changing healthcare through innovations, conferences (TEDxMaastricht 2011, 2012) and lectures, I sometimes meet people who have the ability to bridge the world of medicine and the one of technology on a high and, most of all, broad level. One of those was a young medical student who was running a medical blog (Scienceroll), at that time already the best read blog in this area. Sharing the same vision with a different approach we got connected through the Internet in 2009 and I asked him to speak at our REshape conferences in Nijmegen.

Berci is one of the few people who have the insight, the feeling, the expertise, the tone of voice and the network to guide medicine through this era of change. He's crafted himself a way through huge challenges, carefully choosing his options, staying authentic to changing medicine. Being faculty at Singularity's University in the Exponential Medicine track (formerly known as FutureMed), I asked Daniel Kraft who is running the track, if I could donate half of my lecture

Foreword

time to Berci in 2013. What better place than NASA's Moffet Field campus to show this guy's great competence that equals the levels most of us have at the end of our career; and as expected he absolutely rocked the place. Over time, his opening sentence in his keynotes changed from „I'm a medical geek" to „I'm a medical futurist" and that is spot–on. The question only was how and when he would set the next step. His latest endeavor is the book you are holding right now.

An exciting journey and guide through developments, paradigm shifts, hurdles and opportunities. Although the model of writing a book might become obsolete in the future, it nowadays still is a great form factor to spread knowledge. This book should be added to every curriculum's mandatory reading list in the medical as in the nursing field, but also to every Health MBA program out there. I'm also looking forward to the online course version of this book that he hopefully will create.

In here you'll find a lot of very interesting topics assembled into one place to guide you through your own journey. Since that is Berci's biggest suggestion to you: start NOW exploring the world around you from an innovation perspective, find your own way, and choose your own battle.

My 'prescription' to you would be to read a chapter a day, digest it for another day, explore that area yourself for the day after, and then execute on it the next. But the chances you'll read this book in one take are actually much higher, and that's fine too.

Next to this incredibly well written and overarching book, he's also created a virtual landing space for the discussion on **www.medicalfuturist.com.** I really do hope to meet you there.

To Berci: congratulations my friend, you've done it again! You never stop amazing me and many others with the thorough steps you take. I would like to advise you with an adapted quote of the great Steve Jobs „….keep the courage to follow your heart and intuition… Stay hungry, and be a bit more foolish sometimes…"

Lucien Engelen
@lucienengelen
Director REshape & Innovation Center, Radboud University Medical Center
Chief Imagineer Dutch National IT Institute for Healthcare
Faculty Exponential Medicine, Singularity University, Silicon Valley

Preface

We are facing major changes as medicine and healthcare now produce more developments than in any other era. Key announcements in technology happen several times a year, showcasing gadgets that can revolutionize our lives and our work. Only five or six years ago it would have been hard to imagine today's ever increasing billions of social media users; smartphone and tablet medical applications; the augmented world visible through Google Glass; IBM's supercomputer Watson used in medical decision making; exoskeletons that allow paralyzed people to walk again; or printing out medical equipment and biomaterials in three dimensions. It would have sounded like science fiction. Sooner or later such announcements will go from multiple times a year to several times a month, making it hard to stay informed about the most recent developments. This is the challenge facing all of us.

At the same time, ever-improving technologies threaten to obscure the human touch, the doctor-patient relationship, and the very delivery of healthcare. Traditional structures of medicine are about to change dramatically with the appearance of telemedicine, the Internet full of misleading information and quacks offering hypnosis consultation through Skype; surgical robots; nanotechnology; and home diagnostic devices that measure almost anything from blood pressure to blood glucose levels and genetic data.

People are generally afraid of change even though there are good changes that bring value to all of us. The challenge we are facing now can lead to the best outcomes ever for the medical profession and for patients as well. My optimism though is not based on today's trends and the state of worldwide healthcare. If you read this book you will realize, as I did, how useful technology can be if we anticipate for the future and consider all the potential risks.

Many of us have already witnessed signs of these. Patients, for example, use online networks to find kindred individuals dealing with similar problems. Doctors can now prescribe mobile applications and information in addition to conventional treatment. Given what I have seen over the last few years as a medical futurist, no stakeholder of healthcare—from policy maker, researcher, patient, to doctor—is ready for what is coming. I see enormous technological changes heading our way. If they hit us unprepared, which we are now, they will wash away the medical system we know and leave it a purely technology-based service without personal interaction. Such a complicated system should not be washed away. Rather, it should be consciously and

Preface

purposefully redesigned piece by piece. If we are unprepared for the future, then we lose this opportunity.

According to "Digital Life in 2025" published by the Pew Research Internet Project in 2014, information sharing through the Internet will be so effortlessly interwoven into our daily lives that it will flow like electricity; the spread of the Internet will enhance global connectivity, fostering more worldwide relationships and less ignorance. These are going to be the driving forces of the next years. But without looking into the details, the upcoming dangers will outweigh the potentially amazing advantages.

My background as a medical doctor, researcher, and geek gives me a unique perspective about medicine's future. My doctor self thinks that the rapidly advancing changes to healthcare pose a serious threat to the human touch, the so-called art of medicine. This we cannot let happen. People have an innate propensity to interact with one another; therefore we need empathy and intimate words from our caregivers when we're ill and vulnerable.

The medical futurist in me cannot wait to see how the traditional model of medicine can be improved upon by innovative and disruptive technologies. People usually think that technology and the human touch are incompatible. My mission is to prove them wrong. The examples and stories in this book attempt to show that the relationship is mutual. While we can successfully keep the doctor-patient personal relationship based on trust, it is also possible to employ increasingly safe technologies in medicine, and accept that their use is crucial to provide a good care for patients. This mutual relationship and well-designed balance between the art of medicine and the use of innovations will shape the future of medicine.

This book tries to prepare readers for the coming waves of change, to be a guide for the future of medicine that anyone can use. No one can say what exactly is going to happen and how healthcare will be redesigned, although it is possible to paint a picture of the key directions we are headed in, and act as a "tourist guide" for what kind of skills and knowledge will be necessary to make informed decisions.

I have spoken with global experts about the role that artificial intelligence can play in medical decision making; how surgical robots can assist surgeons; how genomics can make primary care uniquely personalized, and how wearable devices can eliminate the need to go to a clinical laboratory. I have conducted nearly seventy interviews with these experts to augment my own analyses. Through online networks I leveraged the power of crowdsourcing by giving other experts a chance to inform me of trends they find interesting. Experts in medical ethics, for example, helped ensure that individuals for or against extensive technological use find the information and perspectives they are looking for.

Through its stories, descriptions, and suggestions, I hope this guide will fulfill its mission and prepare you for the future of medicine.

Part I. Introduction

"Prediction is very difficult, especially if it's about the future."
-Niels Bohr

In the early 1990s when I was about 10 years–old, I volunteered in computer shops in order to learn about the hardware behind the software. I learned how to construct a personal computer (PC) myself, something I still do these days. As a kid I enjoyed getting access to the newest gadgets and witnessing the continual improvement of computing power.

One day a man in his forties came into the shop and asked about the largest hard drive available that time. When we told him its capacity was 40 megabytes, he asked what he would do with so many megabytes. His operating system, programs, and files would not fill up that much space back then. Today, home computers have terabyte–sized hard drives. As of 2014, the Internet holds approximately 2 zettabytes of information (about ten thousand billion times larger than that man's hard drive). This improvement occurred in just over a decade.

I am lucky to live in an era when technologies are improving at an incredible pace. I remember exactly when I first went online, and know that most of my own students have no idea when they did. On November 21, 1996 at exactly 2 a.m. my computer's modem squealed and as if by magic I was online. I could browse the web if I knew the addresses by heart. Mostly that was it, the whole experience of using the Internet. Eighteen years later I work and sometimes seem to live online in order to experience a world seemingly without limitations. Now smartphones track health parameters and record electrocardiograms (ECG). Artificial intelligence is getting better at diagnosing complicated cases; and augmented reality could let us see more of the online world in real life. I managed to crowdsource a rare diagnosis by having hand–picked experts to follow on Twitter for years. I see how technology can improve the quality of life. Yet new technologies have not really changed the way we organize healthcare.

Even though I passionately love technology as a geek, I know it will certainly not solve the problems that healthcare is facing now. It can facilitate healthcare renovation by providing powerful tools, data, and solutions, but patients need emotional attention and empathy from their caregivers. The lack of connectivity among people and healthcare institutions is a basic problem we struggle with worldwide. I think I might tell my children in 10 years that the early 2010s was a barbaric era because neither physicians nor patients had access to the data they truly needed.

The exponential amount of medical information makes it impossible to be up to date and doctors burn out. Instead of reading a few articles that might be of interest to a particular doctor, let's curate and crowdsource the very best of medical research in a customized way for them. Instead of manually typing data via keyboard, let's speed up the process and make it more interactive through augmented reality. Doing that, the doctor can look the patient in the eye and engage their problems in a conversational manner. There is no smartphone application for empathy and offering emotional care.

Let stakeholders access whatever information they need about a medical condition or its treatment. Let them access public health data that can monitor one's health status and automatically send out customized alerts about advisable changes in lifestyle. Let doctors use this information and devices to provide better care, and let patients use home monitoring services to take better care of themselves. Everyone will benefit.

New technologies will finally help medical professionals focus more on the patient as a human being instead of spending time hunting down pertinent information. They will be able to do what they do best: provide care with expertise. In turn, patients will get the chance to be equal partners in this process taking matters into their own hands.

Let's prepare for what is coming next

I give a lot of presentations every year traveling to many countries. Everywhere I have seen the same kind of system shaped like a pyramid. The base features health insurers, governments, and pharmaceutical companies depending on the country. In the middle of the pyramid are medical professionals bearing almost all the responsibility. These stakeholders sometimes mention patients in the smallest segment at the top of the pyramid. This system has been dramatically changing for years to move the patient to the center and break the pyramid down. The patient will soon be able to measure any health parameter about themselves at home; tell what exactly they eat; record blood pressure, ECG, and other basic data almost constantly.

These patients, now called e-patients, who are ready to hack and disrupt healthcare need to be educated about the use of the digital world as some of them cannot find what they need online, and thus become frustrated,

Part I. Introduction

frustrating their doctors in turn; while others face the problem of too many choices. Moreover, without proper health management taking care of their own health, not only disease; it is going to be impossible to change the structure of practicing medicine as the activity and participation of patients are required for that too.

With a few exceptions medical education has not trained medical professionals for this world full of technological advances. They are trained for today's trends and technologies, while computational power has been increasing at an exponential pace. As futurist Ray Kurzweil has pointed out, these exponentially fast developments might lead to a point where we will not be able to embrace the next logical step. We might create an artificial intelligence that can design algorithms and robots we can no longer understand. I think such changes will lead to even bigger concerns in medicine due to their sensitive nature. Fully automated surgical robots; microchips modeling human physiology, or nanorobots living in our bloodstream all will provide incredible opportunities as well as pose threats.

Evidence based medicine is meant to ensure that quality treatment options are chosen and diagnosis is based on empirical evidence rather than personal assumptions. But this area adapts to changes more slowly than other industries do. For example, after the driverless car developed by Google ran for 1 million miles without incident, car manufacturers such as Volvo announced the inclusion of such algorithms in its future models. For obvious reasons things are a bit slower in healthcare. But soon an ever-increasing gap is going to be too big to cope with.

The most tech-savvy people would agree that the human touch should not be eliminated from practicing medicine; and those who are against technologies must agree that without technology it is impossible to provide healthcare today.

The solution is to prepare patients, doctors, nurses, policy makers, and other stakeholders for the waves of change coming toward us. I remain confident that it is still possible and that we still have time. The goal is to initiate public discussions about the potential advantages and risks we will face.

The role of a medical futurist

In 2012, at the age of 27, I fulfilled my childhood dream by becoming a medical doctor and finishing my PhD in genomics. I was ready to live my entire life as a researcher. But to be honest I was not completely satisfied, and felt unable to leverage the power of my geek self and the technical experience I had gathered. I had to create a new profession in which I could use my different backgrounds and points of views. This is how I became a medical futurist.

The role of a medical futurist is not that of a trend watcher. My interest lies in the intersection of improving healthcare with technology and being a doctor trained for the art of medicine. This gives me both the chance and responsibility to offer my analyses of the future of care.

Early on I received an exciting challenge from a medical journal to summarize the future of healthcare in 2050—and to do so in one Twitter message, in 140 characters. I preferred to write essays, but came up with this: "In 2050, transparent healthcare, decision trees, curated online content, e-patients, web-savvy doctors, and no collaborative barriers."

I'm certain we are heading towards that direction, although without a public discussion initiated now, the chance for establishing a mutual relationship between technologies and the human touch is getting smaller every day.

Part II. Trends That Are Shaping the Future of Medicine

"Don't follow trends, start trends."
–Frank Capra

The hardest part of the job of any futurist, particularly a medical futurist, is picking up the trends, technologies and concepts that seem to play a major role in the future of medicine and healthcare as extrapolations for the next years based on today's trends. What makes it truly complicated is the fact that many of these technologies and concepts intertwine and mix together from many perspectives. The use of artificial intelligence is imminent in the world of electronic medical records, as well as advanced robotics or portable diagnostics.

I chose the topics that appear in the next chapters because they demonstrate the most potential to illustrate what I see as future trends. The goal of these chapters is to give you a clear picture about the key steps being taken in technology by keeping the future of medicine in mind.

The anatomy of a trend description

Each trend's sub-chapter contains basic descriptions about the technology, real-life stories, practical examples, the concepts that determine its use in medicine and healthcare; and possible future directions. Regarding the twenty-two trends, we will move from concepts that are currently available to technologies that are way off in the future.

At the end of each section are scores that meant to give a better understanding of a particular technology's usefulness:

- **A score of availability** between 1 and 10, where 1 is currently too futuristic a concept while 10 means it is already available.
- **Focus of attention** that describes which stakeholder can best take advantage of the trend.
- **Websites & other online resources** that keep you in the information loop by following them.
- **Companies or start-ups** working on the particular trend and being in the forefront.
- **Books and Movies** describing the advantages and disadvantages of the trend or technology.

Trend 1. Empowered Patients

In November in 2013, I was waiting at the airport in Budapest for e-Patient Dave deBronkart. I had invited him to speak at Semmelweis Medical School. Years ago he decided to empower patients worldwide through advocacy, books, and speeches. His experience in tackling kidney and then skin cancer drove him to seek new approaches and solutions.

In January 2007, he was diagnosed with late-stage kidney cancer after a routine shoulder X-ray showed a spot in his lung. It turned out to be one of many kidney cancer metastases all over his body. The median survival time at diagnosis was 24 weeks. Surgeons at Boston's Beth Israel Deaconess Medical Center removed the extensive mess, and gave him a chance to participate in a clinical trial for the powerful interleukin-2 he also read about in online patient forums. By September he had beaten the disease. During his treatment he was in constant contact with his physician, Dr. Danny Sands, one of the earliest proponents of e-patients.

Healthcare cannot really advance without physicians letting their patients help themselves and be a full partner in making the decisions that affect them. This is the key message of deBronkart's book, *Let Patients Help*. After reading it, and reading it again, I sent him a Twitter message that his book should be available to every medical student in the world. He accepted my invitation and flew to Hungary, explaining what he saw as the key problems we have to face during the drive to the medical school.

"A century ago, a patient with diabetes could not know their status without going to the doctor. Today we have home test strips, and sometimes we even have continuous glucose monitors. This has not put endocrinologists out of business; instead, it means we can spend clinic time discussing what to do with the situation, instead of giving part of the time to understanding what the situation is.

You could say that a doctor has many skills: knowledge, diagnosis, prescribing, caring, monitoring, on and on. It is inevitable that some of them will be automated. This is no insult to the physician unless the physician feels they are sacred because "Only I have this magic skill." To me, when some tasks get automated, it creates more space for the skills that remain."

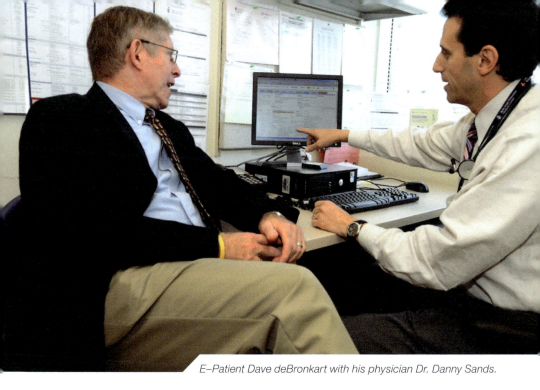

E–Patient Dave deBronkart with his physician Dr. Danny Sands.

He thinks it is possible to make medicine truly patient–focused by ensuring its scientific background while encouraging patient empowerment at the same time. He valued having doctors and nurses who *cared* about him when he was dying and in need of surgery. He now cannot imagine why a smart, caring, and scientifically–minded doctor would not also be able to do the same with a patient who is empowered.

"The only problem I've seen is the rare case where a doctor has been taught to think that the only reason they're valuable is because they know something other people don't know. If that's your self–image, then indeed it's a threat when somebody else knows something. To that, all I can say is that my doctors know thousands of times more than I do, and I love them for it, and I still want to be the best partner I can for them."

He has come across many examples of medical professionals' adoption of digital communication. His doctor, Dr. Sands, is a great and positive example of a physician who wants to be equal partner with his/her patients. deBronkart explained their relationship with a recent story.

Trend 1. Empowered Patients

"A year ago I had just arrived in Switzerland, and I had a worrying symptom in my leg. Did I get a deep vein thrombosis on the flight? We fired up Skype and I used the webcam to show him the ripples on my leg. Boom: he was much better able to assess my situation. He said "Yes, find a clinic," and I did."

In medicine as in other fields, the ability to do our best depends on awareness of the situation, which technology makes infinitely easier from afar. That, in turn, makes it infinitely easier for patients to access care. This is transformational for the provider, whether they want to sell more services or to reach more souls in need.

As deBronkart described, no medical school 10 or 20 years ago was teaching doctors that in their professional lifetimes they would be expected to adapt repeatedly to completely new tools that were unforeseeable. Now that is reality. In his 1987 book, The Media Lab, visionary Stewart Brand spoke of how people would ponder questions like "What could we do if we had unlimited free bandwidth?" This seemed insane in the days of old modems, but today we can see how valid that question was. deBronkart shared with me the three things he looks forward to in the future.

1. Instant dissemination of information where it is needed. That could be by push or by pull (e.g., RSS subscriptions), and includes medical literature and data about any patient's status.
2. A demand for that information, because if people do not know about an opportunity and do not ask for it, then nothing good will come of it.
3. Finally, a layer of analytics that will analyze the data flood and draw our attention to it only in situations that require it.

Dr. Bob Wachter at UCSF Medical Center pointed out that in commercial aviation it became necessary to display less as more and more data poured into the cockpit. In such a world, scarce commodity is not the issue; the viewer's attention is. If that resource is squandered on a flood of mixed–value data, nothing can be optimized. The filter, the analytics, becomes the gate.

Trend 1. Empowered Patients

New online communities

If healthcare already served the absolute needs and rights of patients, there would be no reason for the empowered patient movement to be born. But obviously it is not the case. Patients need to step up in order to reach a relationship with their doctor that is more of a partnership than the traditional hierarchy. Patients in the early 2000s started to take matters into their own hands; launching movements that promote healthy lifestyle and information management; looking for details about their condition to be able to better manage it; and using digital channels and devices to acquire data about their body.

First they started to look for information they had not had access to before. It used to be a privilege of medical professionals. Then they brought the data and information found online to their caregivers, but not all professionals were glad about this. I personally witnessed such cases when the professor left the examination room saying "Well, then you do not need me here" after the patient told him she found information about her symptoms online. This is certainly not the way of assisting patients who want to check online resources. Instead, doctors now need to acquire skills related to digital literacy making them able to assess the quality of a medical website and help their patients in this way too.

Gradually, e-patients have been transforming this approach. They have formed communities sharing insights and details about living with their conditions. I have been in touch with e-patient leaders for many years who have proved that a fellow patient can understand their problems better than any medical professional.

PatientsLikeMe.com was the first widely popular site. It was only open to patients who could log a lot of data about their condition and everyday life. The results of the first research using data obtained through such online communities were published in Nature Biotechnology in 2011 and in the open access paper PLoS Medicine in 2012. In 2014, PatientsLikeMe announced a five-year agreement with Genentech, a pharmaceutical company, to use PatientsLikeMe's global online network to develop innovative ways of researching patients' real-world experience with disease and treatment.

Frustrated patients tend to turn to the Internet for help. Instead of seeking a formal second opinion they try to crowdsource the diagnosis behind their symptoms. CrowdMed.com was designed to serve this special need.

Users can create a case by describing the symptoms and relevant details. For cash rewards medical detectives suggest potential solutions and then collectively vote on the most likely ones. Then CrowdMed's patented prediction market technology aggregates this knowledge to assign a consensus-based probability to each.

There is a personal story behind any true innovation. Carly Heyman, the sister of Crowdmed founder Jared Heyman, was desperately seeking help for a serious condition after contacting nearly two dozen doctors and spending over $100,000 in medical bills. Jared founded CrowdMed to harness the wisdom of crowds to help solve difficult medical cases. Carly's medical case was ultimately solved by collaboration among an interdisciplinary team of medical experts.

Another innovator, Gilles Frydman, played a crucial role in patient empowerment by launching mailing groups for cancer patients and founding the Association of Cancer Online Resources (ACOR) in 1995. These e-mail groups provided patients with a chance to interact with others dealing with the same condition and facing similar issues. ACOR grew to become the largest cancer mailing list ever, and Frydman continued innovating to help cancer patients globally.

I met him several times in locations from California to Paris. He always amazed me with his vision about how we should assist patients in finding the information they need and connecting them to one another. I was not surprised to hear about his new venture, Smart Patients, an online community site that shares details about treatments, clinical trials, the latest science, and how it all fits into the context of an individual's experience.

As a result of these, a new movement was born. The mission statement behind the movement known as Participatory Medicine states:

"Participatory Medicine is a model of cooperative health care that seeks to achieve active involvement by patients, professionals, caregivers, and others across the continuum of care on all issues related to an individual's health. Participatory medicine is an ethical approach to care that also holds promise to improve outcomes, reduce medical errors, increase patient satisfaction and improve the cost of care."

It has its own peer-reviewed journal, provides a forum for collaborative research exchange, educational resources, and advocacy.

Trend 1. Empowered Patients

E–patients are the hackers of healthcare

The term e–patient is derived from attributes such as empowered, engaged, equipped, enabled, equal, or expert. All of these represent the way e–patients disrupt healthcare.

Kathy McCurdy, a designer in her professional life, has been dealing with a neurological disorder for many years. When she had to visit a new doctor she decided to help him by creating an infographic containing years of details about her medications, treatments, operations, and other elements. It gave her new doctor a clear picture and facilitated their working together.

Salvatore Iaconesi from Italy launched a crowdsourcing effort when he found out he had brain cancer. Being a good coder, he cracked the code of his medical records and made the data open source that anyone could analyze. He encourages people to create a video, an artwork, a map, a text, a poem, or a game from the data to help find a solution for his health issue.

In another case, a mother suddenly developed malignant high blood pressure and complex partial seizures after giving birth to her third child. She was treated at Stanford, but received no final diagnosis. Her husband launched a Facebook page to solicit suggestions. He also created a wiki page for listing potential hypotheses so that anyone could easily leave comments. Later they published the graphs of seizure activities and noticed strong and consistent intervals. So many ideas were submitted in their crowdsourcing campaign, that they had to launch another one for finding a method by which this huge amount of data could be analyzed.

Such examples highlight ways patients can obtain a second opinion or assist their own caregivers in solving a complicated issue. As a consequence, more and more start–ups are focusing on this area. Developing services for e–patients, however, is not as simple as it may sound.

I met Jason Berek–Lewis, social media consultant at Healthy Startups, in Melbourne, Australia because I wanted to hear his thoughts about social media and the world of start–ups in healthcare. He has extensive experience working with digital health innovators. We talked about driving forces that shape innovation for start–ups focusing on healthcare.

Trend 1. Empowered Patients

"You can boil most of the factors driving innovation in healthcare into two categories: money/cost/affordability and improving access to healthcare. With Western governments facing major financial challenges together with increasing health costs (driven by technology inflation and aging populations), start-ups and innovators will play a critical role in creating faster, cheaper, better and more accessible ways to deliver essential healthcare services."

Healthcare start-up clones will probably arise, meaning that cost pressures in Western health systems will lead to innovators to look toward other countries' start-ups and adapt their innovations in their local health system.

Berek-Lewis has firm views on what trends seem to be truly disruptive in medicine. One is crowdfunding for healthcare. Some patients will look to crowdfunding to help them to afford access to care and new technologies. Another is increasingly cheaper smartphones and tablets. Asian and African phone manufacturers will continue to drive down the cost of Android-based phones, and the ability of the Android operating system to run on lower specced processors coupled with a backlash against Apple's rumored HealthBook will drive more developers to build for Android first. He also described how hospitals could become the new health start-up incubators. Doctors, nurses, medical specialists, and administrators will continue to push the "bring your own device" boundaries and will work with others to build mobile tech solutions that get around outdated technologies used in hospitals.

With respect to the obstacles that health-related start-ups face in promoting more access for patients, he thinks the Western model is broken.

"The stakes are obviously very high in healthcare; you are potentially 'playing' with people's lives when utilizing new technologies. But trying to reform and change healthcare by doing exactly what we are already doing, and trying to jam this reform into existing and broken models of delivering care, and expecting better health outcomes and more efficiencies is the epitome of insanity. We have to accept that the prevailing Western model of delivering healthcare is broken and free up the regulatory framework (while protecting physician/patient safety) to unleash new opportunities for innovation."

Trend 1. Empowered Patients

According to Pew Internet Research 72% of Internet users say they looked online for health information within the past year. It is partially the responsibility of medical professionals now to assist their patients in learning the meaningful use of social media and the Internet in general. Doctors should acquire the required skills for this. In order to deal with the huge amount of false information online, dynamic resources should be curated by medical professionals and expert patients. On Webicina.com, which I founded, such resources curated by experts are available for free either for patients or their caregivers in over twenty languages. This is the only way to assist all stakeholders.

Today's hierarchy of the patient–physician relationship will dramatically change to create a system in which the patient is in the center of attention. They can measure anything about themselves; access information and resources without limitations, manage their health or disease, and take equal part in making medical decisions with their caregivers. Examples of how healthcare is being transformed include patients buying companies that go bankrupt conducting clinical trials so that they can continue the trials themselves; and patients launching their own companies to help others. The movement is still only taking baby steps. It is just the beginning.

Score of availability: 10
Focus of attention: Patients
Websites & other online resources: E-Patients (http://e-patients.net), Patient Opinion (https://www.patientopinion.org.uk)
Companies & start-ups: SmartPatients (https://www.smartpatients.com), CrowdMed (https://www.crowdmed.com), ACOR (http://www.acor.org), Patientslikeme (http://www.patientslikeme.com), Webicina (http://www.webicina.com)
Books: Let Patients Help by E-Patient Dave deBronkart; The Complete Guide to Managing Health Care Using Technology by Nancy B Finn
Movies: Extraordinary Measures (2010)

Trend 2. Gamifying Health

Do we currently have health care or sick care? Do we care more about disease or health? All of us know how hard it is to keep ourselves in shape, have a healthy diet, and live a healthy life. Gamification seems to be the key in persuading people to live such lifestyles or stick to the therapy they have been prescribed to. Over 63% of American adults agree that making everyday activities more like a game would make them more fun and rewarding. Wearable gadgets, online services, games, and mobile health solutions can lead to better results if gamification with the right design is included. Improving our health or making our job more efficient can and therefore should be fun.

Since the age of 14, I have been logging details of my life every single day. It means not one day is missing from my digital diary which now consists of over 6,600 days with data. I have logged how much I slept; the major things I worked on; and a physical, mental, and emotional score from 1 to 10. Based on that, I have been able to make significant decisions about my lifestyle as I could always check my health data when I changed an element in my diet, habits, or exercises. It has been a tremendous help. I use Withings Pulse, a small tracker, to measure my daily physical activities and the quality of sleep; and I play on Lumosity.com for 5 minutes every day to constantly improve cognitive skills that I use in my personal and professional lives.

The grandmother of Mike Scanlon, Co-Founder of Lumosity, was diagnosed with Alzheimer's disease, and he saw how devastating it was. While a neuroscience PhD candidate at Stanford University, he came across advancements in brain research that never made it out of academic settings. He wanted to make those results and methods available for the general public. That was when Lumosity was born. By playing games online every single day, our short- and long-term memory, flexibility, attention, and focus can be improved.

A study conducted by the University of Washington found that performance on Lumosity games can distinguish between patients with cirrhosis of the liver, pre-cirrhotic patients, and healthy controls. In that study Lumosity games were used as psychometric tests to detect subtle cognitive impairments. Such gaming solutions will be immensely implemented in future research and even clinical trials.

The movement of making lifestyle-related decisions based on everyday measurements of health parameters is called "Quantified Self".

Trend 2. Gamifying Health

Patients facing the same medical problem such as sleep issues gather around a table and discuss the potential underlying reasons, bad health habits, and ways to improve their sleep. Then they measure the outcomes, collect as much data as possible, and then assess the success of the methods they agreed upon. By incorporating technology into data acquisition about aspects of a person's daily life from mood and diet to physical activity it has been leading the way for gamified solutions in healthcare. People everywhere can now easily measure health habits and parameters every day, compare data, share it with others and make informed choices.

Gadgets and devices that can measure fitness, sleep, and even blood glucose levels have started to flood the market. It is becoming hard to choose the right one. Amazon.com has recently launched its wearable technology marketplace where different tools can be compared to each other based on several parameters.

By making more social applications, the Quantified Self has recently started to transform into the "Quantified Us" movement. Imagine that with the right data, anyone could tell why they had an awful sleep last night, or what the reason was behind the last seizure for a patient with epilepsy. The opportunities are endless and there are only a handful of obstacles to overcome such as the quality of the logged data, or the potential overuse of these gadgets.

Persuading people to follow therapy

WellaPets is a smartphone application that can be downloaded for free on the App Store, Google Play or Amazon Appstore. The child adopts, customizes and begins caring for his or her own Wellapet. By regularly visiting their pet, kids are able to play games with them, collect items for their pet's home, and care for their pet's asthma. Developers have worked with pediatricians to ensure that Wellapets teaches kids what they need to know if they, their friend or their sibling has asthma.

I discussed the use of gamified applications with Alexander Ryu, the Co-Founder and CEO of LifeGuard Games, Inc. who took leave from Harvard Medical School to launch his company.

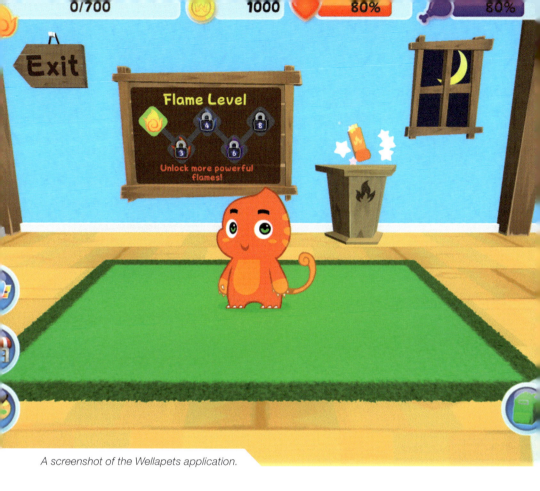

A screenshot of the Wellapets application.

"We have seen Wellapets improve the way clinicians connect with children by helping clinicians speak kids' native language, through games. Wellapets helps clinicians replace jargon and often-somber topics with a more playful and understandable medium for teaching kids how to stay well. We have also seen that the social nature of games helps foster dialogue between kids, talking about health and wellness in a way that feels normal and free of stigma."

Although he thinks that gamification is not the right term for what they actually do. Fun and good game design should be consistently prioritized over educational objectives or behavior change strategies, because perfect educational content serves little purpose when a game is not fun enough to hold a user's attention. Speaking from experience regarding early prototypes of Wellapets, Ryu describes that gamification unfortunately implies taking a concept that is not a game and applying some magic treatment that turns it into a game which is fundamentally the wrong approach to designing quality games.

Trend 2. Gamifying Health

The ultimate goal according to Ryu is healthcare payers accepting such technological alternatives at least as much as traditional medical services given the fact that these can improve health outcomes in a significant way.

Gamification expert and author of *The Gamification Revolution*, Gabe Zichermann, said that fundamentally people are bad at deferring pleasure now for future gain and avoidance of pain. Games are designed to help raise people's engagement in a way that is more powerful than what we have seen before.

Even, companies tend to realize the power of gamification and use it in keeping their employees healthy. According to Gartner, an information technology research and advisory company, more than 70% of the world's largest 2,000 companies are expected to have deployed at least one gamified application by the end of 2014. Keas, an employee health and wellness program in the United States, integrates gamification with biometrics devices to motivate employees at large enterprises to engage in health and wellness activities. Moreover, using personal health data, it can identify risks and suggests actions that can be taken to manage those risks. In the near future, being a good worker might not be a good enough reason to be kept in your job, but being healthy will be an additional requirement.

An example of health–related gamification is "stick" developed by Yale University economists. Users create so–called commitment contracts that bind them to a specific goal. Users define goals such as losing weight or learning new languages. They can add incentives such as putting money at stake. They can designate a referee to act as a third party and they can add supporters to help them reach their goals.

"MySugr Companion Diabetes Management App" works as a diabetes logbook providing immediate feedback and rewarding users with points which can be used to tame their "diabetes monster". The goal is to tame the user's monster every day, thus keeping track of their medical condition.

A New York–based company, Kognito, developed "Start the Talk", an educational, role–playing game to help parents talk about underage drinking with their kids. Players develop conversational strategies to approach, educate, and build trust with their kids about drinking.

"Run an Empire" typifies the group of apps that use alternate reality. It challenges users to conquer territory and defend it from rivals through actual physical activity. "My ASICS" is a smartphone app serving as a mobile monitor that personalizes running based on current stamina. The smartphone application "Zombies, Run!" requires the runner to pick up virtual supplies and

Trend 2. Gamifying Health

escape from virtual zombie hordes. It is an ultra-immersive running game and audio adventure, delivering the details of zombies attacking the city into the user's headphones. By using augmented-reality devices such as Google Glass, runners can actually see the virtual zombie hordes added to the real life scenario.

Video games and platforms in the hospital

Years ago, I had a chance to receive a few copies of the "Re-Mission" video game and distribute it to local pediatric clinics. Children fighting cancer loved the 3D shooter game. They could play through 20 levels that took a character on a journey through the bodies of young patients with different kinds of cancer while shooting at cancer cells and bacteria with an arsenal of weapons and super-powers: chemotherapy, antibiotics, and the body's natural defenses. The color of the pills they shot at the cancer cells could actually resemble the ones they took in real life. A study of 375 cancer patients concluded that playing "Re-Mission" led to more consistent treatment adherence, faster rate of increase in cancer knowledge, and a faster rate of increase in self-efficacy in young cancer patients.

Other video gaming platforms offer different opportunities. The controller of Nintendo Wii is different from the controllers of other video game consoles as it can be held with one hand and uses technology that senses the player's movements. The Wii has been used in studies to measure its effectiveness in neurocognitive rehabilitation or in the treatment of Parkinson's disease. Retirement and nursing homes use Wii to motivate their residents to be more active by imitating the movements of bowling or tennis with the controller.

The Microsoft Kinect 3D sensor is able to monitor and analyze performance in real time, giving patients feedback as they exercise and complete assignments. By playing interactive games that use motion-reading sensors, doctors can track up to 24 points on a patient's body. The Kinect is used to promote healthy lifestyle and fitness; manage physical therapy and rehabilitation, facilitate virtual visits by medical professionals, and even screen young children for autism spectrum disorders. An Israeli company called BioGaming developed a cloud-based platform that lets physical therapists and trainers create personalized exercise routines that are automatically transformed into interactive, engaging games.

Skills acquired while playing video games have been proven useful in training surgeons, because using new surgical instruments requires similar skills. Laparoscopic or minimally invasive surgery that lets surgeons perform operations in the abdomen through small incisions demands fine movements, while surgeons watch the camera's view on screen instead of looking at their own hands. In one experiment surgeons who had a history of playing video games for more than three hours a week made 37 percent fewer mistakes and completed tasks 27 percent faster than the surgeons who had no history of playing video games. Several medical schools such as the University of Washington now advocate teaching surgeons these skills through similar games in clinical settings.

Sticking to a therapy is hard

Adherence or compliance, the degree to which a patient correctly follows medical advice, raises crucial issues in improving health and decreasing the cost of healthcare. An estimated 50% of patients with chronic diseases do not follow the prescribed treatment. The economic burden of this is evident.

Several start-ups have targeted this issue with different solutions such as a pill bottle that glows blue when a medication should be taken, and red when a dose is missed while alerting family members at the same time. In another example, tiny digestible sensors can be placed in pills and transmit pill digestion data to physicians and family members. Proteus Health develops such digestible sensors which transmit the pill's identifying signal with the exact time of detection to a smartphone or other Bluetooth-enabled device. It even includes an accelerometer. Don Cowling, the company's senior vice president, told about a man in California who can track whether his father with Alzheimer's disease, who lives in a nursing home in the United Kingdom, has taken his medication. He can also see how his father sleeps at night. Online health tracking has gone to a new level.

In the future, it is going to be extremely difficult not to fully comply with the prescribed therapy patients agreed upon. Moreover, compliance with medication should be as simple and comfortable for patients as possible. The real goal is to be able to measure health parameters, monitor them and engage when needed. As it is nearly impossible to get everyone motivated about their own health, let's find solutions that trick them into that by implementing methods of gamification seamlessly into their lives.

Trend 2. Gamifying Health

What if it became common to track our health parameters and get alerts when something goes wrong? People could get rewarded for living a truly healthy lifestyle by getting access to premium services or wellness facilities for lower fees. Gamifying our health could facilitate compliance and teach children how to cope with a chronic condition. Gamification might be the key for a broad range of issues for which we currently have no good solutions.

Score of availability: 6
Focus of attention: Patients more than medical professionals
Websites & other online resources: Amazon's Wearable Technology database (http://www.amazon.com/b?node=9013937011), Games for Health (http://gamesforhealth.org/ and http://www.gamesforhealtheurope.org/)
Companies & start-ups: AdhereTech (http://www.adheretech.com/), Proteus Digital Health (http://www.proteusdigitalhealth.com/), Wellapets (http://www.wellapets.com/), My ASICS (http://my.asics.co.uk/), Re-Mission (http://www.re-mission2.org)
Books: The Gamification Revolution by Gabe Zichermann
Movies: Believe in Gamification! (Short Film – http://youtu.be/ziHCvpikLh8)

Trend 3. Eating in the future

Many of the innovative technologies presented in this book will fundamentally change not only the way we consume food but also food itself. Today, getting access to clean water and basic nutrients is a constant battle in several parts of the world; while obesity and non-healthy diets place an economic burden on the society in developed regions.

The world population is expected to surpass the 9 billion milestone by 2050. Estimates by the Food and Agricultural Organization suggest that demand for meat will more than double over the next 40 years. Traditional livestock methods will struggle or fail to meet this demand, and the challenge to keep people healthy will get more complicated. The culture of eating and producing food therefore must change.

As a potential solution for global food shortages, companies have been experimenting with 3D printing, although most 3D food printers can only print basic foodstuffs that require only one to six ingredients. The ultimate goal is to print out complete customized meals on demand. In the movies "Back to the Future II" and "The Fifth Element," delicious dishes were constructed in seconds by putting the ingredients into a special oven. Today Foodini, a project introduced on the crowdfunding site Kickstarter, aims at printing out food using fresh ingredients. It can make ravioli, cookies, or crackers. The instrument's food capsule must be filled with fresh ingredients, and the recipe has to be inputted. In caseds where the ingredients are pre-cooked, the food is ready in a few minutes' time.

Jeff Lipton, a researcher who develops 3D printed food at the Cornell Creative Machines Lab, in Ithaca, NY, said that most innovation is aimed at overturning the status quo, with the focus on either making food production more efficient or more customized. This is the direction the food industry is about to look at.

Another example of how 3D printed food could ease our lives is the use of 3D printers in nursing homes. Plenty of nursing home residents suffer from dysphagia characterized by the inability of the larynx to close properly while swallowing, causing renal failure, pneumonia and even death. Purified food could be a solution. Because meals are important social events in nursing homes, and it can be frustrating to look at the delicious plates of other residents, the smoothfood concept was born. It is about deconstructing and reconstructing fresh food to smoothfood which looks equal to the original.

Trend 3. Eating in the future

In a new project to be finished in 2015, 3D printers will help create food that can be easily swallowed and looks great at the same time. According to Matthias Kück, chief executive of Biozoon, when residents bite on the reconstructed food, it is very soft, and practically melts in their mouth.

Stem cell burgers and the world's healthiest food

A few years ago, growing hamburger meat from the muscle tissue of a cow would have been the perfect basic story for a documentary about the future, but now it is possible to do so. It started nearly 20 years ago when NASA got approval from the United States' Food and Drug Administration (FDA) to begin developing meat for use during long-term space missions. In 2008, People for the Ethical Treatment of Animals (PETA) announced a prize of $1 million to anyone who could create stem-cell derived chicken meat. To date there is still no winner of the prize. For years, environmentalists and animal

Jellified chicken wing with carrots and potato mash printed out by Biozoon.

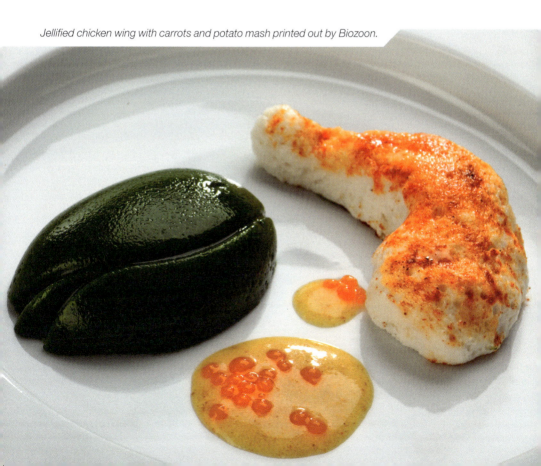

Trend 3. Eating in the future

rights activists, among others, have been awaiting a commercially-viable alternative to conventional meat using stem cells. The final product is referred to as "schmeat" because it grows in sheets and the cells remain flat while differentiating into muscle tissue.

The Cultured Beef project aims to make commercially available meat created by harvesting muscle cells from a living cow. It is incredibly efficient as it uses 99% less space than modern livestock farming; moreover, cells from a single cow could produce 175 million quarter-pounders while traditional farming methods would need 440,000 cows for that. Raising livestock takes a tremendous amount of food, water, and energy; additionally, the methane produced in the gastrointestinal system of the animals is adding to greenhouse gas emissions. According to a recent estimate, lab-grown or "in vitro" meat has the potential to reduce energy consumption by 45%, greenhouse gas emissions by 96%, and land use by 99%. Imagine the economic and logistic advantages of switching to this new method. Of course, the technique is not ready for mass production, and the taste is still an issue.

The taste of "stem cell burgers" is not like what we prefer today, but it will likely improve at the same exponential rate as computing power did over time. Currently, the lack of naturally-occurring fat in schmeat requires that fillers and substitutes be used. By 2020, though, we might not be able to differentiate burgers made by traditional means and those created by this new method. In 2013, Mark Post of the University of Maastricht in the Netherlands hosted probably the world's most expensive barbecue in London, inviting two food critics and one chef to try the schmeat burger. Each serving cost about $385,000. The test-tasters concluded that the burger's texture was good, but the patty was not really juicy.

Lab-grown meat does not benefit from the animal's natural immune system that keeps harmful micro organisms away; therefore the use of antibiotics in the production process of the schmeat is another issue that needs to be addressed. Conventional livestock consumes 80% of all antibiotics sold in the United States and this should not be an example to follow.

The 1968 movie "2001: A Space Odyssey" showed astronauts consuming very simple-looking food that contained all the ingredients the body needs on a long space mission. Recently, Rob Rhinehart invented Soylent to make this concept real and widely available. He looks forward to the point where instead of being an obligatory function to stay alive, eating food can be art.

Soylent is a beige-colored beverage that Rhinehart claims contains every nutrient the body needs. It was named after the ubiquitous food substitute in the dystopian science fiction movie, "Soylent Green." After raising $3 million from investors, and testing the product on himself and a few volunteers, Rhinehart believes it is ready to be commercially available. Soylent ingredients are open-sourced and classified by the FDA as "generally recognized as safe."

For months Rhinehard has consumed nothing but Soylent every day. He plans to get the cost down to $5 per day for a diet yielding 11,000 kilojoules or 2,600 kcal. Some newspapers such as The Telegraph sought comment from academics about Soylent, but they were so skeptical about it that they declined to be interviewed. Other experts expressed surprise that anyone would want to replace real food with a synthetic mixture. They also underlined the importance of the many micronutrients in fruits and vegetables that cannot be exactly replicated in a formula. Even if Soylent were formulated properly and individuals could live on it, these nutritional experts doubted they would experience optimal health.

While it not might be the ultimate solution for hunger globally, it shows the way where researchers are heading.

Do you know what you eat?

It might surprise you that right now we can only assume to know food ingredients based on the short descriptions printed on food cans and packages.

One solution might be provided by TellSpec, a hand-held device designed to determine what macronutrients or specific ingredients the food contains using spectroscopy which is the study of how wavelengths of light change when reflecting from various surfaces. Isabel Hoffmann, founder and CEO of TellSpec, ran a successful Indiegogo campaign that raised $386,392 in 2013. I asked about her personal views and vision. As usual, there was a personal story behind this novel idea.

Hoffmann, a serial entrepreneur, started several software, Internet, and healthcare companies before moving to Canada in 2011. Only three months after arriving in Toronto, her 13 year-old daughter became really sick. She experienced a series of allergies, angioedema (swelling of the subcutaneus tissue), and anemia (a decrease in the amount of oxygen-carrying hemoglobin in the blood). Medical professionals thought it was a viral infection that would

Trend 3. Eating in the future

get better on its own. But it did not. She dropped out of school. Hoffmann stayed at home taking care of her daughter. At times the girl's blood pressure became so low that she couldn't walk to the bathroom. Hoffmann happened to come came across a book by Dr. Neil Nathan in which he offered hope to those whom the medical system had been unable to help. She took her daughter to Dr. Nathan who diagnosed the girl with severe penicillin allergy and an array of food allergies. As a result of this episode Hoffmann began to meet other people suffering from similar problems.

Her goal then became to help people who must avoid toxic foods, and those who have to watch their diets closely but cannot be sure of what they are actually eating ingredient by ingredient, allergen by allergen. She found the right people, created a concept, and finished the crowdfunding campaign in 2013. She shared with me what happened after the campaign.

"A group in Brazil tries to deal with the epidemics of obesity among Brazilian Indians due to the fact that now they have access to processed food. There are challenges related to obesity and famine we have to face now. We don't really know what we eat. Regarding environmental diseases, the number one exposure is the skin; while the number two is the gastrointestinal system therefore what we eat is crucial. Technology finally got to a stage where people can really benefit from that. Between October and November in 2013, we received 20 000 e-mails."

The two directions TellSpec is heading in at the moment are genomics; and establishing a spectrome, a database of how the wavelength of reflected light changes depending on the surface characteristics of the object illuminated. The direction she wants to head in is truly personalized medicine.

Hoffmann, a TED Global speaker in 2014, envisions a bright future of portable diagnostics. She described, for instance, a wristwatch device that would integrate TellSpec data with that from the genome and the microbiome (the genetic fingerprint of the microbe colonies that live in our gut). With such a device people could make decisions based on real-life data. They could know what breakfast should be on a given day based on these data. They would have power, knowledge, and information that we are missing now in our society.

New devices are meant to make sure we eat the right food with enough nutrients and in the right way. Examples include HapiFork, an electronic fork that vibrates when the user eats too fast. It also helps monitor

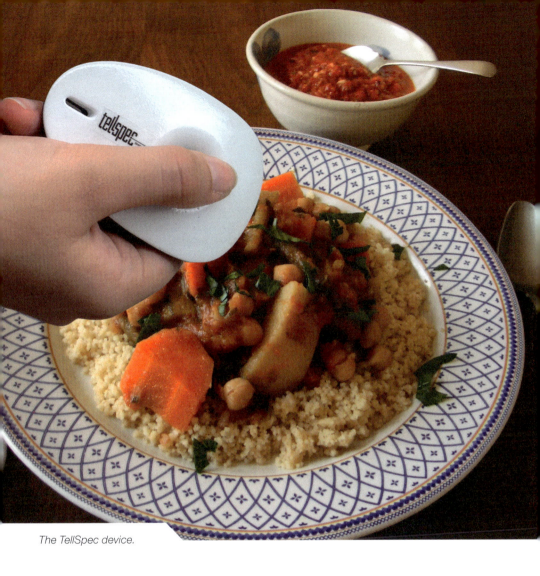

The TellSpec device.

and track eating habits. For example, it tracks how long it takes to eat a meal, the amount of "fork servings" per minute, and how long the intervals are between fork servings. Like many others I cannot find enough time to eat. The HapiFork taught me how to slow down, although it is embarrassing to know how fast and how incorrectly I used to eat every day.

Other ideas with the potential to transform the way we eat could include smart knives. Besides measuring the levels of nutrients such as sugar, vitamins, protein and fat in the food that it cuts, such a smart knife could also check levels of harmful bacteria and pesticides. It might emit negative ions to help keep the food fresh. A Spanish company has invented food tattoos: a laser can safely etch logos and even QR codes onto fruits and vegetables.

Trend 3. Eating in the future

Amazon's new smartphone can scan and recognize almost any product, including food items, and direct users immediately to the relevant website. Augmented reality can help people stick to a diet: researchers in Tokyo used a visual headset to make food look one-and-a-half times bigger, which led to a 10% decrease in consumption.

For many decades human populations around the globe have not been able to deal with the nutritional opposites of obesity and famine even though our knowledge about the optimal diet has dramatically increased over the same time. Futurist Ray Kurzweil and nutritionist Dr. Terry Grossman described a futuristic concept in their popular book, *Fantastic Voyage: Live Long Enough to Live Forever*. They would eliminate the need to actually eat food by using nanorobots that would transmit the right amounts and types of nutrients to each of our cells. Future people would wear a "nutrient belt" loaded with billions of nutrient-laden nanobots that would enter and leave the body through the skin as needed.

A thorough review recently concluded that technology will increasingly change the way we interact with food and drink. It will facilitate our interaction with and knowledge of what we consume by enhancing entertainment value, providing diners with targeted multisensory interventions, and providing alerts or nudges to those who may wish to eat in a more healthy way. There is a risk of technology becoming a distraction to diners, possibly resulting in an unwanted increase in food intake or the emergence of bad habits. It depends on us.

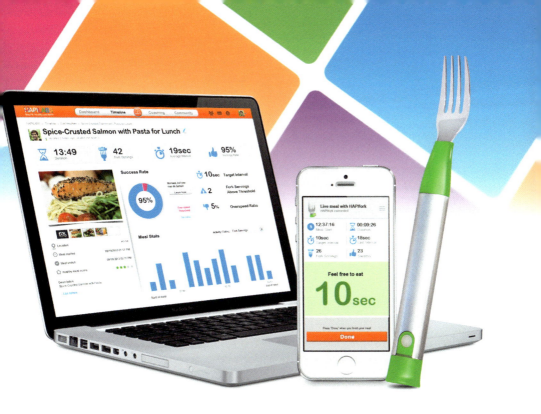

The HapiFork device, application and web portal.

Score of availability: 3
Focus of attention: Consumers
Websites & other online resources: The Future of Food (http://food.nationalgeographic.com), European Learning Partnership About The Future of Food (http://fof.gaiaysofia.com), Personal Blog of Bill Gates (http://billgates.com/about–bill–gates/future–of–food).
Companies & start-ups: Soylent (http://www.soylent.me/), Hapi (http://www.hapi.com/), Tellspec (http://tellspec.com/)
Books: The Prince's Speech: On the Future of Food by Prince Charles; Can We Feed the World? by Conway
Movies: Soylent Green (1973)

Trend 4. Augmented Reality and Virtual Reality

Augmented reality (AR) is a real-time view of a real-world environment that is enhanced by computer-generated sound, video, graphics, GPS data, or inputs we may not have thought about yet. Imagine wearing an AR device while you are walking, and receiving promotional offers from shops you pass. Simultaneously you see the real and online worlds superimposed. A company called Metaio, for instance, provides an AR application for technicians to service and repair the Volkswagen XLI without any prior training. Instructions are projected on top of what they are looking at in the auto shop. Getting information via a Google Glass or digital contact lenses could greatly augment the practice of medicine.

Google Glass, a wearable computer with an optical head-mounted display, was made available to testers and developers in 2013. As of July, 2014, it is not yet commercially available, although Google did sell it publicly for one day in April, 2014. Google Glass has a touchpad on the temple piece, a camera, and an optical display. It works like a smartphone by letting users take photos and videos, browse the web, take notes, and make calls. Wearers access the Internet via natural language voice commands such as "OK, Glass, do a search for diabetes".

Dr. Rafael Grossmann, a Venezuelan surgeon living in the US and also a good friend of mine, woke me up late at night in June 2013. He was about to become the first surgeon to demonstrate the use of Google Glass during a live surgical procedure. I got out of bed and followed his operation sitting at my computer. It was a fantastic proof that AR is advancing, and that one of the areas most likely to benefit from it is medicine.

Dr. Grossmann noted that students used to learn while looking over the surgeon's shoulder. Now he can demonstrate what he is doing much better, and to hundreds of students at a time because his point of view can be projected onto huge screens. Stanford medical doctor, Dr. Abraham Verghese, started using Google Glass because he can make videos of patient examination for medical students to watch from his own point of view.

Dr. Grossmann gave a presentation at one of the most beautiful places in Central Europe, Lake Balaton, at a congress organized for young surgeons. He described how difficult it has been to maintain eye contact with the patient during an office visit when he had to repeatedly turn to his computer and input data. Even with the subsequent spread of tablets, he

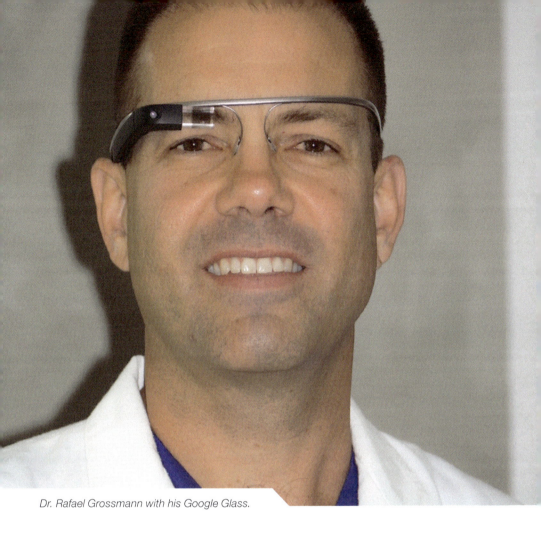

Dr. Rafael Grossmann with his Google Glass.

still had to look down at a screen. With Google Glass, eye contact is steady. Being able to always face the patient creates a much better ambiance and doctor–patient relation.

    Lucien Engelen, director of the ReShape Innovation Center at Radboud University Medical Center, The Netherlands has studied using Google Glass in clinical settings since 2013. His focus has been the quality of pictures and videos, the opportunities for remote consultation, how checklists can be displayed to the treating physician, and even the device's battery life. While there are many potential benefits in a healthcare setting, Engelen concluded that technical issues currently make using the device complicated and limited.

    In the near future laypersons could save lives if the basics of cardiopulmonary resuscitation were displayed on the Glass. The app could be launched with the simple voice command "OK, Glass, CPR." An algorithm

Trend 4. Augmented Reality and Virtual Reality

developed by Hao-Yu Wu and colleagues at the Massachusetts Institute of Technology (MIT) demonstrated that an ordinary cell phone camera can detect a person's pulse with accuracy. Building on this, Glass might be able to tell if an individual who has collapsed has regained a pulse or not. Imagine a case where it detects no pulse: the Bee Gees' "Staying Alive" starts up and guides the user to perform chest compressions at a 100 beats per minute. The motion tracker embedded in the Glass could determine if the compressions are adequate, and the accumulated number of compressions would be tracked. At the same time the device summons an ambulance to the exact GPS coordinates and sends send text messages to the nearest hospitals with information about the situation so they can prepare.

With Google Glass, a clinician could look at the lines on a test strip used with blood or urine, and receive back the correct yes/no results as well as quantitative measurements—all within seconds. In the future, the strips are marked with individual QR codes to make this possible in everyday clinical settings.

Glass could let patients quickly get in touch with a medical professional who would see what the patient is seeing from their point of view. In Melbourne, Australia a company called Small World teams up Google Glass with the Australian Breastfeeding Association. It allowed their telephone counselors to see through the eyes of new mothers as they struggled to breastfeed at home.

Another project initiated at the Rhode Island Hospital in the US used Google Glass in the Emergency Room to remotely connect with a dermatologist whenever their expertise was needed.

Since December 2013, doctors used Google Glass at Boston's Beth Israel Deaconess Medical Center to see whether it can facilitate either doctor-patient interactions or the input of data. Huge QR codes hang on the walls and doors of patient rooms. These can be scanned when the doctor steps into the room, and Glass transmits the relevant patient records and information. Doctors can keep eye contact with the patient while receiving pertinent information right away. In April 2014 Google Glass scanned through the entire history of a patient and revealed that that person had given incorrect information. As a result the doctors could save his life.

In another case an Emergency Room doctor was dealing with a patient with a massive brain bleed. Google Glass automatically pushed the patient's allergy history and current medical regimen into the doctor's field of vision. It gave him critical extra time to reverse, time he might otherwise have spent turning away to a laptop or notepad.

I had a chance to see a Google Glass AR application called MedicAR in action. Looking at a specified image through the camera of Glass, a 3D anatomical model appeared just like in real life.

Dr. Christian Assad-Kottner and colleagues published the first paper on using Google Glass in medical education. It concluded that wearable technology has the potential to enhance medical education and patient safety once widely available. The authors recommended that medical institutions should develop policies that address patient privacy when using technologies to enhance medical care.

In a parallel development, the Alvin J. Siteman Cancer Center announced the development of high-tech glasses to help surgeons visualize cancer cells. Live ones glow blue when viewed through the eyewear. First used during surgery in February 2014, the device helps distinguish cancer cells from healthy ones and also lessens the number of stray tumor cells left behind. While the technology is certainly not a 100% accurate at detecting each types of cells, the glasses could potentially reduce the need for additional surgery and spare patients from stress and expense.

Layar remains one of the best-known and most frequently downloaded augmented AR browsers for smartphones. With over 35 million downloads to date, it was one of the first apps to demonstrate the potential of AR. In a joint project with the ReShape Innovation Center in Nijmegen, The Netherlands, Dutch citizens can see exactly where semi-automatic defibrillators are located by using Layar on their smartphones. In an emergency the camera in the phone guides them to the closest device. Similar apps could be used with AR glasses or contact lenses.

Have you ever had a bad experience when a nurse had trouble finding a vein when attempting to take a blood sample? Success doing this is purely based on experience. Being able to spot an available vein would make this process more convenient and less painful. A new wearable, Eyes-On™ Glasses, uses imaging technology to find the location of the most suitable vein. The device is readily used in physician offices, clinics, and hospitals.

The success of such a technological breakthrough depends on the quality and quantity of applications available for the specific device. To help start-ups focusing on using Google Glass in healthcare join accelerators and incubators, Palomar Health and Qualcomm Life teamed up to build an incubator for developers called Glassomics.

Trend 4. Augmented Reality and Virtual Reality

The launch of the prototype already raised ethical and privacy concerns. What happens, for example, with private data when Glass is lost or stolen? How does the public react to the knowledge that it can record videos any time? Motorists have been reportedly pulled over for driving while wearing the Glass. Las Vegas casinos have banned the use of Google Glass even before its release. These examples show how far we still are from implementing it in practice.

From glass to contact lens and beyond

In one of his talks in 2013, Babak Parviz, an electrical engineer at the University of Washington, proposed using contact lenses for continuous body monitoring. Given that contact lenses are used by more than 100 million people, it is a good candidate for a continuous sensor. Lenses could contain miniature glucose sensors, for example, along with readout circuits and an antenna. Such a system could remotely powered by radio frequency broadcast, making it wake up, take a measurement, and send the data back before powering itself down.

Eyes–On™ Glasses on a nurse.

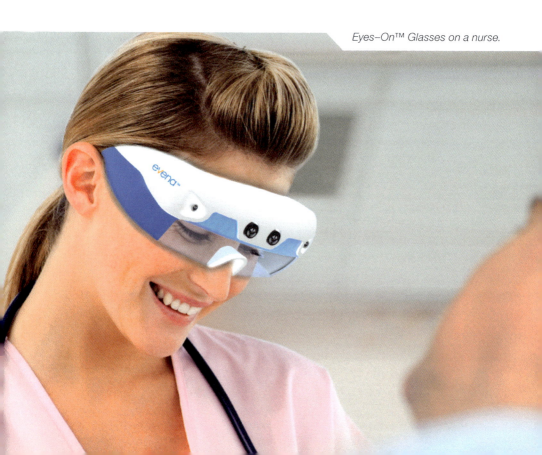

Trend 4. Augmented Reality and Virtual Reality

Google Glass can be controlled through voice and hand gestures. In the future contact lens sensors would be controlled with brain waves. Given developments in this area, the idea is quite plausible. The potential leveraging power of AR is huge enough that medical professionals should address patient privacy first, and justify its use in practice with evidence.

Lenses made of graphene, a special form of carbon, could make possible the manufacture of smart contact lenses, or ultra-thin devices whose infrared camera would extend users' vision to spectrums that are not visible to the human eye. Moreover, future contact lenses will not only allow us to look into a world augmented with additional information, but might also constantly measure and log health parameters.

According to the US Patent & Trademark Office, Google is working on a multi-sensor contact lens that would work with Google Glass, other wearables, Android smartphones, smart televisions, Google Now, and similar devices. By blinking, it will enable a user to turn the page of a book or proceed to the next song. Ultimately, it may be possible to insert a screen into the lens. But this will take years to fulfill.

Eventually hardware will probably not be needed to add data. Screens and keyboards will be projected on the wall or on a table, making it straightforward and accessible anywhere in clinical settings. Holographic keyboards hovering in front of the user will next make us forget about smartphones and tablets. The data will be stored only in the cloud. Small devices will probably replace personal computers and laptops, and not need traditional accessories such as keyboard and mouse. With ultra-high definition video streams and 3D binaural audio, online consultations will sound like real life. Gesture-sensitive interfaces similarly to those seen in the movie "Minority Report" will make interaction with big data commonplace. With virtual reality and increasingly sophisticated holograms, the practice of medicine will be re-invented.

New diseases resulting from excessive use of virtual reality (VR) in gaming and business can be expected. For example, virtual post-traumatic stress disorder (v-PTSD) which occurs in gamers wearing VR masks who participate in enormous virtual battles such as "Call of Duty." Their symptoms may be exactly the same as those in soldiers who fought in real wars. On the positive side, VR could be employed in psychotherapy. People will be able to virtually visit distant places or other worlds that they would never be able to experience in real life. Anxious patients could go through an upcoming operation step-by-step, or choose a hospital based on its "virtual experience" package.

Trend 4. Augmented Reality and Virtual Reality

Popular and intensive VR applications might induce some people to live their lives in the virtual world. The popularity of Second Life, one of the earliest VR environments online, decreased over time because it could not improve on the experience. But what if VR chambers become commercially available, allowing users to feel the world while sitting at home in a chair? They might live an entirely digital life, shop, meet others, and even work in an artificial environment. How would these possibilities change society? What could we do to persuade people not to switch from real life to a virtual world?

The first bi-directional brain-machine interfaces allowed monkeys to use a brain implant to control a virtual hand and also get feedback that tricks their brains into feeling the texture of virtual objects. Building on this, an Ottawa-based company called Personal Neuro is exploring the possible benefits of Google Glass analyzing the electrical activity of the brain, the electroencephalogram (EEG). We might not be far from controlling wearable devices with our thoughts.

Using such solutions in the operating room would take medical specialties to the next level. Currently, surgeons use cautery in which an electrical current heats tissue to make incisions with minimal blood loss. The intelligent iKnife goes one step further by analyzing the vaporized smoke by mass spectrometer to detect what molecules are in the biological sample. Doing so, it can identify in real-time whether the tissue is malignant or not. There is no need to send a biopsy specimen to the pathology lab.

A clinic in Germany started experimenting with a tablet-based AR application. During operations, surgeons can perform more precise excisions because they are guided by the patient's radiology images, which lets them see through anatomical structures.

Opportunities are almost endless. With the development of Google Glass, Sony's Morpheus, and Oculus Rift which was acquired by Facebook in 2014 for $2 billion, medical applications will likely expand in the coming years. After being sold to Facebook, the Oculus Rift team predicted that over the next 10 years, virtual reality will become ubiquitous, affordable, and transformative. There is still time to live up to these expectations.

Trend 4. Augmented Reality and Virtual Reality

Score of availability: 4
Focus of attention: Medical professionals more than patients
Websites & other online resources: GlassOmics (http://glassomics.com/), Google Glass applications (http://glass–apps.org/)
Companies & start–ups: Evena Medical (http://evenamed.com/), Google Glass (http://www.google.com/glass/start/)
Books: The Google Glass Revolution by Samuel Cole; Augmented Reality: An Emerging Technologies Guide to AR by Kipper & Rampolla
Movies: The Terminator (1984), Predator (1987), Minority Report (2002), Iron Man (2008), Avatar (2009), Surrogates (2009)

Trend 5. Telemedicine and Remote Care

Hugo Gernsback was a pioneer in both radio and publishing. He designed the first home radio set and published dozens of magazines in the early 1900s. He wrote an article about the future of radio telecommunication in the February, 1925 issue of Science and Invention. The device was the "teledactyl" (tele means far, dactyl means finger in Greek) and was meant to allow doctors to see and touch their patients through a viewscreen with robotic arms that was kilometers away. He predicted that the practice of medicine would look much different by the 1970s. From their offices doctors would diagnose and treat patients in their homes via machines and devices that worked through radio waves. He described the device in details.

"The doctor of the future, by means of this instrument, will be able to feel his patient, as it were, at a distance. The doctor manipulates his controls, which are then manipulated at the patient's room in exactly the same manner. The doctor sees what is going on in the patient's room by means of a television screen. Every move that the doctor makes with the controls is duplicated by radio at a distance. Whenever the patient's teledactyl meets with resistance, the doctor's distant controls meet with the same resistance. The distant controls are sensitive to sound and heat, all important to future diagnosis."

The idea of the teledactyl demonstrates how the doctor–patient relationship could take place at a distance. Actually, the first complete tele–surgical operation using a surgical robot was performed by a team of French surgeons located in New York on a patient in Strasbourg, France over a distance of several thousands of kilometers in 2001. It was called the Lindbergh operation named after American aviator Charles Lindbergh who was the first person to fly solo across the Atlantic Ocean. From one perspective, partial loss of the human touch is inevitable. But medical practice does not have to go entirely digital. When there is already an established relationship between patient and the doctor, a digital interaction can save time and effort for both parties.

From another perspective, the shortage of doctors is global. Solving this will require extensive use of digital methods. In the United States alone, the shortage of doctors is predicted to rise to 130,000 from the current 60,000 by 2025; and Africa has 25% of the worldwide disease burden but only 3% of the

Trend 5. Telemedicine and Remote Care

health workers. It is almost impossible to train all the physicians that will be needed.

To tackle this iRobot and InTouch Health announced in 2013 an autonomous remote-presence robot called RP–VITA. The FDA cleared its use in monitoring surgical patients before, during, and after their operations. It cannot perform remote operations given that it has no manipulating appendages, although extendable pan, tilt, and zoom lenses could allow collaboration between a remotely-located surgeon and one on site. Such a device could travel autonomously to destinations where doctors are in short supply.

Acute Care RP–VITA® by InTouch Health.

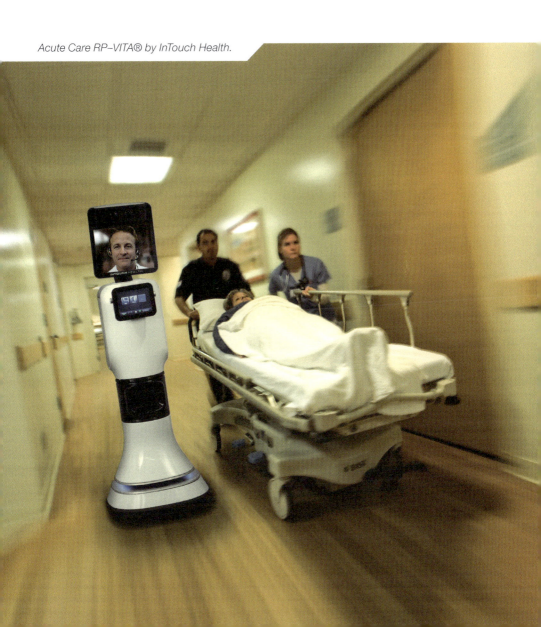

Trend 5. Telemedicine and Remote Care

Dignity Health in the US uses similar video–conferencing machines that move on wheels and project the physician's face on a large screen. These robots have cameras, microphones, and speakers. According to Alan Shatzel, medical director of the Mercy Telehealth Network, the robot can be at the bedside in minutes no matter where the patient is located. For the physician operator, it feels like being with the patient in the room. Nothing can replace in–person care, but as Shatzel described, it is the next best thing.

For the last century illness triggered the same scenario. The doctor was summoned; he arrived at the house and made a quick assessment; and then he either prescribed a therapy or admitted the patient to the hospital. Telemedicine may prompt the first real change when a doctor is available only through online channels and a webcam. In the not–too–distant future telemedicine could evolve to generate a holographic image making the doctor's presence in the patient's home almost real. Only the remote touch remains to be worked out.

In the video game industry, a concept called force feedback has been used since the 1990s that lets users feel wobbles when driving on rough terrain in a car racing game. In California, I had a chance to use an educational device that simulated taking a biopsy. The force feedback let me feel the skin resistance when I administered a virtual injection. Glove–based feedback systems already exist to give users a remote sense of touch.

House calls of the 21st century

In its 2014 e–health report Deloitte called e–visits the house calls of the 21st century. It predicted over 100 million electronic visits globally in 2014, saving more than $5 billion comparing to the cost of in–person doctor visits. It saw 2014 as an inflection point when costs, quality of care, advances in telecommunications, and professional attitudes would drive their adoption. Their message to policy makers worldwide:

"As e–visits are proven and adopted in the developed world, and as the necessary infrastructure is deployed in the developing world, they are likely to offer affordable primary medical and diagnostic care to very large populations that do not have access today."

Trend 5. Telemedicine and Remote Care

In 2010 the Hawaii Medical Service Association, the state's largest health plan covering over 700,000 citizens, was the first insurer to make the online resource of American Well available to its members. Those insured had the chance to talk with a doctor via a web camera. The remote doctor could send notes to the local one who might be unavailable. Individuals who were not members of the health plan could still use the service on a for-payment basis.

HealthTap is a service where patients pose a question to a panel of doctors. The initial query is free; follow up questions incur a charge. The site claims to have served more than 1.3 billion individual questions and saved over 13,000 lives. Commenting on the service, the American Medical Association warned that Internet should "complement, not replace, the communication between a patient and their physician." It pointed out that online health portals do not take a history, conduct a physical exam, or monitor the suggested treatment. Using such information in isolation could pose a threat to patients.

Some large corporations have tried to develop telemedical services. In November 2013, Google launched Google Helpouts as a successor to Google Answers. It let experts charge clients per session, per minute, or both; with Google initially to take a cut of 20%. Inasmuch as improving telehealth is a Google priority it waived its 20% fee for all healthcare related questions, and ensures that its video interchanges are compliant with HIPAA (Health Insurance Portability and Accountability Act).

Years ago, Maayan Cohen discovered that her healthy, young boyfriend had brain tumor. She found herself sitting in waiting rooms with stacks of papers that created confusion and a feeling of lack of control. Had she received all the results of tests, drugs, treatment, and medical history? Around this time Maayan met Ziv Meltzer, who was suffering from stomach pains no doctor could diagnose. They understood each other perfectly, left their jobs, and launched Hello Doctor, an online service and mobile application designed to manage and make sense of medical records.

Ziv Meltzer explained the background of HelloDoctor to me. In the company, everyone is a patient. The more patient information they collect and can share, the more they can help. HelloDoctor now focuses on collecting, organizing, and managing medical records because for many people that is where the greatest the pain is.

Video consultation is becoming a routine part of care offered by the Stanford Hospital & Clinics. Patients can schedule video visits through the hospital's website; provide information in advance; and at the appointed time

Trend 5. Telemedicine and Remote Care

meet with the doctor in a web-based videoconference from a computer equipped with a webcam.

While the number of similar services continues to grow, there is a need for a connection hub for doctors and medical records. In 2005, Ryan Howard saw a need for affordable, easy-to-use technology that met the needs of small medical practices. Howard quit his job, sold his car and house, and launched Practice Fusion. Before he had been in a serious motorcycle accident and in massive debt, but decided to use the settlement cash from his accident to pay the salaries of three employees. In 2014 the company has more than 110,000 medical professionals and handles more than 80 million patient records.

The ultimate goal of gathering big data in electronic medical records (EMR) ¬managed by professionals, and personal health records (PHR) updated by patients is creating smart alerts in natural language. That is, the system would understand the actual meaning of words and expressions in the records, thereby making it simpler to intervene in a patient's affairs when needed.

At the TED 2014 conference in Vancouver, Canada, Larry Page, CEO of Google gave an interview in which he mentioned electronic medical records years after Google Health, the company's early effort, was shut down. He said we could save a hundred-thousand lives this year if people would share the information of their medical records with the right people in the right ways.

Such innovations try to bring healthcare services to the patient's home. Examples include the HealthSpot station, which looks like doctor's office in a box. It is a telehealth system intended for large institutions and features medical diagnostics, face-to-face dialogue, and electronic health records with privacy. By sitting inside the box, patients can send information related to a physical examination through different kinds of cameras.

Medtronic, the largest medical device maker in the world, develops and provides insulin pumps, glucose monitors, and heart devices that can transmit patient data to a secure server. For diabetes, they eventually want to provide a patient's entire care team with continuous real-time glucose therapy information to avoid life-threatening high or low glucose conditions.

Microsoft has used all its main health and communication products to transform its Kinect device into a telehealth tool for physical therapy by combining the motion-tracking abilities of the Kinect, Skype, and Microsoft's cloud-based HealthVault EMR. Patients see exactly what they should do during their physical therapy session. Results are uploaded to the cloud, and session efficacy can be logged and shared.

Trend 5. Telemedicine and Remote Care

These kinds of devices and services serve to connect patients to doctors when in-person care is not possible. Wouldn't this be a milestone? Patients should be able to download their own medical records. Medical professionals should be able to communicate and consult with each other without limitations. Everything seems to indicate that medical expertise as well as laboratory tests will soon be accessible from home. Due to the shortage of doctors worldwide and the lack of access to medical care in underdeveloped regions, connecting patients to physicians online will receive more and more attention. Telemedicine encourages patients to take more responsibility for their own care; but it does not mean the end of the doctor-patient relationship or personal contact. It should be considered an additional element that makes the relationship even more effective.

Score of availability: 8
Focus of attention: Patients
Websites & other online resources: International Society for Telemedicine & eHealth (http://www.isfteh.org/), The American Telemedicine Association (http://www.americantelemed.org/)
Companies & start-ups: In Touch Health (http://www.intouchhealth.com/), American Well (http://www.americanwell.com/), Practice Fusion (http://www.practicefusion.com/home.php)
Books: Telemedicine and Telehealth: Principles, Policies, Performance and Pitfalls by Darkins & Cary; Connected Health: How Mobile Phones, Cloud and Big Data Will Reinvent Healthcare by Ranck; The Creative Destruction of Medicine by Topol
Movies: Logan's run (1976)

Trend 6. Re-thinking the Medical Curriculum

I graduated from medical school in 2009. Looking back at my time as a medical student, I mostly used relatively old-fashioned books and anatomical atlases. In my later years I began to discover useful social media channels and online resources as well. It was hard to study anatomy and similarly difficult subjects by traditional means. Considering the various solutions and tools that could be useful in medical education nowadays, I do not know how I managed with only printed books.

The medical curriculum is supposed to train students to become healthcare professionals, and prepare them for practicing medicine. The problem is that the medical curriculum worldwide, almost without exceptions, focuses on today's technology and how doctors should deal with today's patients. But both technology and the general needs of patients change quickly.

Usually it takes 4 to 6 years to become a doctor, and another 5 to 10 years to become a specialist. Trying to remember what the world looked like 4 or 6 years ago I recall no widespread use of smartphones, tablets, Google Glass, social media, or artificial intelligence. That is how much the world can change in a few years' time. The rate of change is even faster now. Current curriculum does not prepare students for these even though new applications and technologies are becoming a crucial part of the medical profession. It is time to change and actually re-think the basics of what we call medical education.

As a first step, I launched a course at the University of Debrecen in 2008 that focused on meaningful and safe use of social media for medical students. Since then, the course has moved to Semmelweis Medical School in Budapest, Hungary, and been fully enrolled. The course covers the use of search engines, Facebook, Twitter, Youtube, blogs, and more in a medical setting. We are preparing students for the digital world. My teaching motto is "If you want to teach me, you first have to reach me". When students filled online surveys about their digital habits, and it turned out all of them used Facebook, I launched a Facebook challenge in the form of a page where every day I posed questions about the topics covered in the lectures. Students could compete for bonus points during the semester. It has been a huge success according to students.

The knowledge imparted in this course is called digital literacy. After I presented my experience with this curriculum at Stanford Medical School, a physician based in London wanted to visit Budapest once a week during the

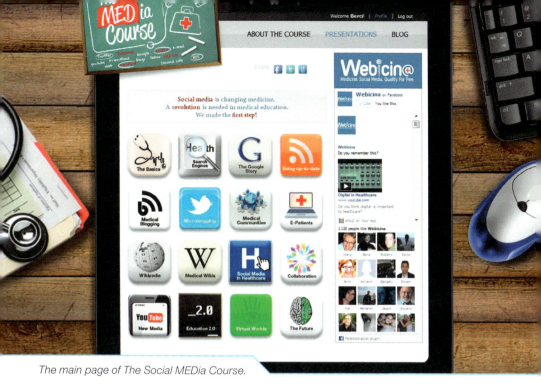

The main page of The Social MEDia Course.

semester in order to take the course in person. There was nothing similar in the United Kingdom. It was the final sign that underscored the need for an online course that would present topics in detail; include hand–outs, study guides, and references; and a test with gamification pertinent to each lecture. This is what I created in 2012 under the name The Social MEDia Course. Since then, thousands of students and doctors (more of the latter than students), started the course. Hundreds acquired the "Ultimate Expert" badge and certification. But it is not enough to focus only on social media and mobile health. We need to prepare students for the world they will face when they actually start practicing medicine. In 2014, a pilot course was launched at Semmelweis Medical School with the mission of giving students a set of skills with which they will be able to navigate the sea of new technologies and the ocean of medical information. Called "Disruptive Technologies in Medicine," this course introduces them to personal genomics, telemedicine, 3D printing, regenerative medicine, imaging health, robotics, and artificial intelligence.

    Such initiatives should be welcome by all medical schools in order to let students acquire skills that were not important before but they will have to use while practicing medicine in the near future.

    Besides these prospective changes, there are numerous reasons why being a medical student should be a good experience nowadays. Online

Trend 6. Re-thinking the Medical Curriculum

networks dedicated to focused topics on Twitter, Google+, Facebook and the blogosphere are capable of many things: filtering the most relevant news when network members trust one another; help crowdsource complicated clinical/scientific questions; create learning groups without geographical limits; and give access to global experts and projects.

The typical curriculum requires students to study texts and data by heart without proper reasoning and understanding the logic behind it. Instead, study through serious diagnostic games has clear advantages. The "Healing Blade" card game takes the player into a world of sorcery and creatures where real–world knowledge of infectious diseases and therapeutics play a pivotal role in the winning strategy. "Occam's Razor" is a real diagnostic card game released by NerdCore Medical. The company also releases Manga Guides to physics, statistics, and biochemistry. It successfully crowdfunded a game on Kickstarter surpassing the original goal of $25,000 with $98,113. The "Bacterionomicon" is an artbook bestiary based on the characters of the "Healing Blade." It has entries for 41 "Lords of Pestilence" covering infectious

Cards about characters representing bacteria and antibiotics in the game of NerdCore Medical.

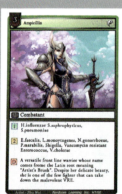
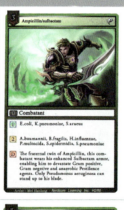
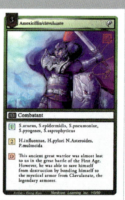
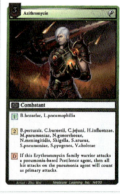
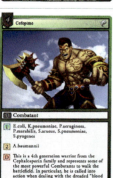
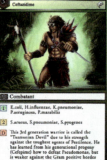
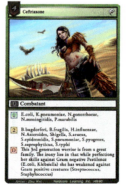
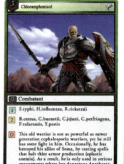

Trend 6. Re-thinking the Medical Curriculum

bacteria, and 27 "Apothecary Healers" representing antibiotics.

It has never been so easy to gather required information in an automatic way. Subscribing to medical RSS feeds; checking news on Feedly.com or PeRSSonalized Medicine (perssonalized.com); setting up automatic Google Alerts (alerts.google.com) for different search queries; receiving peer reviewed papers from Pubmed.com by e-mail; and following citations by Google Scholar (scholar.google.com) have all become effortless, efficient ways of filtering an ever-increasing amount of medical information.

New resources started to appear to facilitate student learning. I had a chance to try The Anatomage Table at the Singularity University, and wish I could have used it in medical school. It is an anatomy visualization system on a human-sized screen for educational purposes, and it is being adopted by many of the world's leading medical schools and institutions. This virtual cadaver combines radiology software with clinical content that lets users visualize any anatomical structure from any angle.

BioDigital Systems recently introduced a virtual human body as a web-based platform with the intent of providing a searchable, customizable map of the human body. John J. Qualter from the New York University School of Medicine helped design the 3D installation. He describes it as a living digital textbook.

The University of Arizona College of Medicine announced an exclusive collaboration between the medical school and SynDaver Labs, a Florida-based company. The company has been producing synthetic cadavers that have a heart that beats and pumps blood, and a liver that can make bile. It has also created the world's most sophisticated synthetic human tissues and body parts. It could simultaneously assist students and reduce or eliminate the need for live animals, cadavers, and human Standardized Patients (the latter are actors trained in a script).

Without doubt, the future belongs to interdisciplinary innovations. For example, neurosurgeons at the University of California, San Diego School of Medicine and UC San Diego Moores Cancer Center use magnetic resonance imaging (MRI) guidance for delivering gene therapy directly into brain tumors. This way, the rest of the brain remains unaffected and the risk of the procedure is minimized. Another company, MRI Interventions, has developed and is commercializing systems to enable minimally invasive procedures under real-time MRI-guidance. The ClearPoint system for real-time, MRI-guided minimally invasive brain surgery is FDA-cleared, CE-marked, and currently

Trend 6. Re-thinking the Medical Curriculum

installed in 29 hospitals. It is being used for direct drug delivery, laser ablation, and drug delivery for patients suffering from Parkinson's disease, dystonia, epilepsy, brain tumors, and more.

Specialists look at the same medical problem from different angles. Because current medical education encourages specialization, social media and other digital technologies can help bring about new ways of collaboration. Combining knowledge from multiple specialties and with computing could result in optimal outcomes for patients.

It is time to re-create the basics of the medical curriculum and re-think how we train future medical professionals who should be not only web-savvy and tech-savvy, but also have the skills to navigate an exponentially changing world of medical technology and information. Their primary goal of treating patients with empathy means that a well-designed balance is needed.

How to design a new curriculum

Some say that medical education has not really changed since the last paradigm shift in 1910 when the Flexner Report, a book-length study of the state of medical education in the US and Canada, advised medical schools to raise their admission and graduation standards, and stick to the protocols of mainstream science in teaching and research. Students today still have to become professionals who care for their patients; are able to collaborate with other disciplines and ancillary caregivers; are creative and critical thinkers; and are motivated to grow constantly as life-long learners.

I had a long talk with Jur Koksma, Assistant Professor at the Radboud University Medical Center, about these issues and the future of medical curriculums when I was a PhD opponent during a thesis defense in the Netherlands.

At Radboud University Medical Center, they are currently working on a revolutionary new medical curriculum. The educational vision behind this transformation has been inspired by people all over the world who want to improve people's lives through healthcare and education. It is based on two pillars that Koksma described.

"First of all, we want to bring students and patients together in realistic learning environments. Students should be 'learning professionals' who start learning by doing from the very first moment they enter the

curriculum. On the very first day students will talk to patients and hear their stories. This way, patient stories will set the narrative in motion that is a doctor's education. Students take genuine responsibility in professional practice, and after such shorter or longer periods of immersive learning, reflect on those practices and on their own competency and related professional learning goals. This is the didactic backbone.

The second pillar besides professional, practice based learning is the didactic principle of self directed learning. Students, as learning professionals, take responsibility for their own learning paths. They organize and manage their own education and, within certain boundaries, get to decide on the contents of their program. In that sense we try to maximize opportunities for personalized education, giving each and every person a chance to become the best doctor they can be on the basis of their unique talents and motivations. We are getting rid of a one size fits all approach in patient care. Let's also do this in medical education."

In this system, each student has a personal coach. They work with a so-called open space technology in which students themselves decide what will be addressed when students and teachers meet. Currently, biomedical and medical students also work as consultants for pharmaceutical companies in an attempt to come up with innovative ideas. These young students still have a lot to learn, but it seems they learn very quickly when under pressure.

Future medical schools will make global digital classrooms possible. The quality of different curriculums should be balanced given the wide access to information and educational resources online. No old books, no cadavers pickled with formaldehyde, no lack of information or educational resources should be issues that future medical schools have to face. Students will train collaboratively with other healthcare professionals, mirroring the cross-disciplinary approach that will be integral to the clinical environment of the future. Enhanced technology will allow for more efficient referrals, faster consultations, and more thorough transitions of care. As a result, providers can spend more time nurturing a strong relationship with their patients. Digital platforms, from IBM's Watson supercomputer to wearable devices, will take part in training students from day one.

Being a successful doctor is not a sprint race, but a marathon. The current examination systems do not really address the skill sets today's medical professionals should acquire. A better option might be to let students advance

Trend 6. Re-thinking the Medical Curriculum

at their own pace and be examined when they have mastered the material. The Clayton Christensen Institute for Disruptive Innovation in San Mateo, California calls this competency-based learning, which is tailoring an educational program and curriculum for each student. If course materials are available online, students can be assessed individually. Knowing when a particular student is likely to perform to his or her full potential on a given exam might be attainable only by analyzing the student's answers with artificial intelligence.

As a whole, the curriculum must be able to address current needs and the ever-changing skill set needed for medical professionals to provide excellent care and use innovative technologies at the same time. It will be a struggle, but never in the history of education have we had so many opportunities to take the medical curriculum to the next level.

Score of availability: 4
Focus of attention: Medical students
Websites & other online resources: The Social MEDia Course (http://thecourse.webicina.com/)
Companies & start-ups: Nerdcore Medical (http://www.nerdcoremedical.com/), Anatomage (http://www.anatomage.com/), Pocket Anatomy (http://www.pocketanatomy.com/), Osmosis (https://www.osmosis.org/)
Books: Medical Education for the Future by Bleakley, Bligh & Browne; Understanding Medical Education: Evidence, Theory and Practice by Swanwick
Movies: The Doctor (1991)

Trend 7. Surgical and Humanoid Robots

Ever since I was a kid I have been constantly improving cognitive skills from speed to focus by using video games. I have tried almost all gadgets. I was therefore not surprised at how easy it was to use a daVinci surgical robot. At the 2013 Futuremed course in California I grabbed the joystick controls, stepped on the pedals, and looked into a viewfinder at a three-dimensional, high-quality image sent back by multiple cameras. I could move around tiny objects gripped by miniature but precise robotic arms.

My instructions for what to do exactly came from Dr. Catherine Mohr, the Director of Medical Research at Intuitive Surgical, and an expert in the fields of robotic surgery and sustainable technologies. She was standing behind me watching what I actually did on a screen. I told her about this book, and she found the time to share her views with me. The reason why I wanted to include her stories in this book is not only her knowledge and experience in this field, but also her similar ideas about technical developments for improving healthcare.

"In the fall of 2013, I was asked to partake in a debate at the Oxford Union. The proposition was "this house believes that the technology revolution will solve the global healthcare crisis". As a physician and a technologist, people were very surprised that I was arguing in opposition to this statement. But although I am a true believer in technology, and the power of technology to transform health care, I firmly believe that technology is a tool in our hands, and that the future of medicine will be humans wielding those tools wisely."

The history of robots and digitization in medicine does not go back very far. An early IBM 650 computer was used to scan medical records for subtle abnormalities in the 1950s; the first computer-assisted program for radiating brain tumors called the Gamma knife was introduced in 1974; the daVinci surgical robot system was launched in 1999; and the Robotic Arm Interactive Orthopedic System for use in partial knee and total hip surgery was introduced in 2004. Since then, development has been extraordinary.

Now, surgeons can control robotic arms and other functions on a control panel in the operating room or remotely through a transatlantic connection. The attention of the surgeon is an obligatory feature in robotic-assisted surgery. The equipment is designed to enhance the skill and experience of human surgeons.

Trend 7. Surgical and Humanoid Robots

Fully automated surgical robots have not yet arrived. Dr. Mohr has considered the issue of autonomy in the use of future medical robotics.

"Robots generally imply autonomous or semi–autonomous motion and decision making, and many of the devices that we think of as robots in medicine and surgery are instead "telemanipulators". With a telemanipulator, the physician's and surgeon's movements and judgment are being implemented through an electromechanical intermediary, but the human remains firmly in control."

The daVinci system, called Xi©.

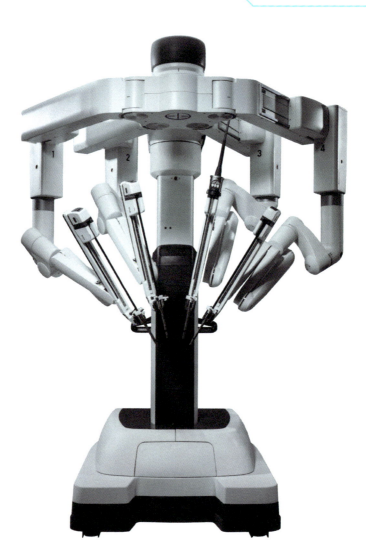

The new version of the daVinci system, called Xi, was released by Intuitive Surgical in 2014. It was designed to allow four-quadrant access to the abdomen, making workflow much easier for surgical procedures such as colorectal surgeries. The scope can be moved from robotic arm to arm, changing the surgeon's point of view without having to re-dock the robot. This allows the surgeon to move back and forth easily in a much wider surgical field than has been possible before. This capability will open up many more areas of general surgery to robotics, and allow more patients to get minimally invasive surgeries. It is even getting less invasive with the adoption of the single incision platform option.

Other areas for improvement include making the scale of operation smaller so that manipulations that are on the edge of a surgeon's capability become more comfortable and precise. Fluorescence imaging is another application. Blood vessels, lymph nodes, and the bile duct can be clearly delineated with dyes that fluoresce under ultraviolet light, making it helpful in many types of surgeries.

Obstacles for wider adoption

One of the obstacles to the wider adoption of surgical robots that must be overcome is correcting the perception of robot autonomy. People are justifiably nervous about surgery performed by a pre-programmed device. They are afraid of the idea of a robot being in control. Consider the case of current orthopedic robots where the cutting paths are predetermined. The robot either executes the plan or provides a haptic guide to the cutting, but a human surgeon is responsible for the planning. The patients are less apprehensive given that they perceive a human in control, not a machine.

Another obstacle is misunderstanding of the economics of robotics. According to Dr. Mohr, people look at the cost of a technology and assume that it simply adds to the cost of doing a procedure. This leads to the perception that robotics raise healthcare costs without adding value equal to or greater than that cost. In reality, robots are enabling surgeries that were formerly done through big open incisions to be done through tiny ones. And while the cost of the technology adds to the cost of the surgery itself, the decreased hospital stay, reduced complications, and lower rates of readmission lead many hospitals to save far more money with the use of the technology than they spend on it.

Trend 7. Surgical and Humanoid Robots

Another challenge facing any company bringing new technology into the healthcare field is regulatory. Regulatory agencies must strike a careful balance between promoting and protecting the public health. When promotion is emphasized, new technologies and drugs with the potential to improve patient well-being are enthusiastically adopted at the real risk of letting some technologies through that turn out to have negative effects. When protection is emphasized, new technologies are assumed to be bad until proven advantageous, and fewer new innovations survive the regulatory process. For a proper balance between promotion and protection, society needs a mature relationship between risk and benefit.

I discussed the potential of using advanced robotics in medicine, as well as the obstacles that must be overcome with Professor Blake Hannaford, Director of the Biorobotics Laboratory at the University of Washington. He worked on the remote control of robot manipulators at NASA's Jet Propulsion Laboratory; was awarded the National Science Foundation's Presidential Young Investigator Award; and is considered an expert of surgical biomechanics and biologically based design of robot manipulators.

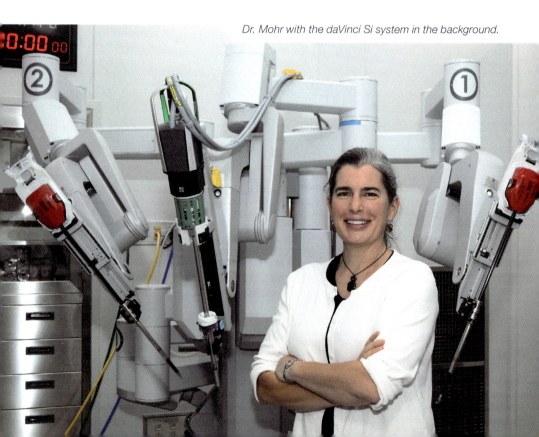

Dr. Mohr with the daVinci Si system in the background.

"As with all medical devices, there is a rigorous trade-off between innovation because of technical possibilities and the duty to apply the most proven methods to each patient. Wider adoption of medical robots requires advances on both fronts. In the clinic, we need to find and validate applications in which the patient has a better and safer outcome with robotic assisted treatment. On the engineering side, we need advances on software architectures for reliable integration of robotic algorithms with teleoperation."

When we talked, he was particularly excited about a project funded by the National Institutes of Health at the Biorobotics Laboratory. In collaboration with the Fred Hutchinson Cancer Research Center they aim to make tumors fluoresce when labeled with a molecule extracted from scorpion toxin. More fluorescence imaging agents will be available on the market soon which would make it simple to see directly where the cancer is and help surgeons avoid nerves and blood vessels.

They also work on developing a robust developers' community that promotes the use of open-source software that is now used at eleven universities worldwide. It is not known how open-source software will flow through the regulatory system, but the FDA is studying the attractive idea that bugs in open-source software can be found and repaired more easily than in software developed by large companies shielded with numerous patents. Researchers think that developing a clear regulatory framework for open-source medical software, including hybrids of open- and closed- source software, as well as longitudinal studies of new robotic assisted procedures that show clinical benefits are much needed to strengthen the power of advanced robotics in the operating room.

An important goal is to feel what the robot touches, which means getting useful haptic feedback from the patient tissues to the surgeon's hands. According to Professor Hannaford, haptics technology has matured a lot in the last ten years, but still struggles to find a robust market niche. Haptic feedback from surgical robotics is in great demand, and will be available eventually. It is still not clear, however, how to certify haptic feedback as completely safe and stable. In the future, surgeons might sit in special chairs, receiving a clear, three dimensional picture of what the robotic arms see in detail, thus be able to control tiny movements in great precision from a distance. In underdeveloped regions, surgical robots could be deployed so that operations are performed by surgeons who control the robots from thousands of kilometers away.

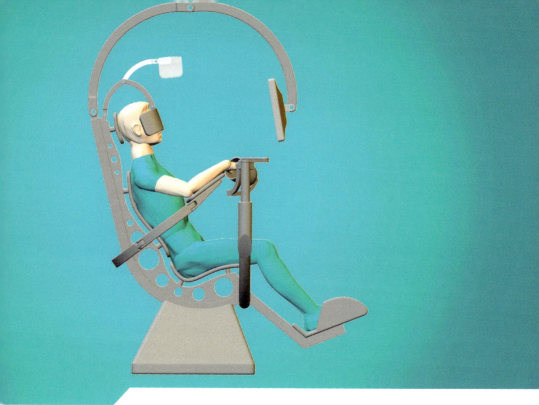
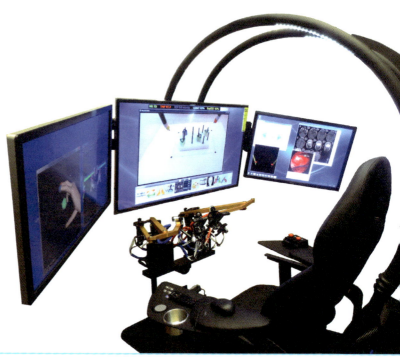

Concept art and a prototype of how future robots with telecommunication systems could be used by medical professionals.

In a chapter he wrote in Medical Devices: Surgical and Image Guided Technologies, Professor Jacob Rosen at the University of California, Santa Cruz, identified three trends which may lead to a revolutionary breakthrough in surgical robotics. First is an effort to reduce invasiveness, which will minimize trauma to surrounding tissue, reducing the risk for infection, and result in speedier recovery and shorter hospitalizations.

The second trend is improvements in visualization. Endoscopic cameras, along with new imaging modalities, provide a view and representation of anatomical structures.

The third trend concerns the level of automation and how much surgeon control is needed to execute the surgical procedure. In 2007, a research program called "Trauma Pod" funded by the Defense Advanced Research Projects Agency (DARPA) demonstrated that the operating room can be fully automated without the need for actual human presence. The surgeon directed the surgical robot via telepresence; the sterile nurse was replaced by a tools changer, an equipment dispenser, and a robotic arm, whereas the circulating nurse was replaced by an information technology system that tracked the tools and supplies used throughout the procedure.

Understanding the value of robotics

Dr. Mohr thinks that even with robotic manipulators, the operating room will never be fully robotic. There are so many tasks involved in keeping a patient stable during surgery that there is little value in building a robot for tasks that humans do better and with great versatility. Humans outdo robots in many areas, and will certainly continue to do so when versatility and adaptability is required.

The cost effectiveness of including new services and technologies like robotics in everyday healthcare is still not clear to anyone but a hospital Chief Financial Officer. While both patients and physicians tend to value technology and embrace it when it leads to better outcomes, neither patients nor physicians in the US healthcare system have access to data regarding the cost side of the equation. It is therefore very difficult to make cost effective decisions such as those Dr. Mohr described. In recent years she has seen the rise of the educated patient who advocates for himself and asks for minimally invasive or robotic surgery. Many procedures happen to be cost effective, but motivated patients still have little understanding of the economics.

Trend 7. Surgical and Humanoid Robots

By understanding surgical robots more, it will be apparent that they enhance the surgeon's capabilities rather than replace them. Such robots can potentially lend a surgeon dexterity, vision, and navigational guidance that are beyond what is possible by the unaided human. Like other cases of disruptive technology, understanding that the surgeon is still in control will go a long way toward easing the public's uneasiness about robotics.

According to these experts, there is huge value in making devices smaller than a millimeter in diameter. Containing robust moving parts, they would move into micro-scale manipulations while still being strong enough to interact with tissues. The ultimate goal that Dr. Mohr shared with me is to get better, more accurate, and early diagnosis of cancer so that we can operate when they are surgically curable. Achieving this could make cancer a speed bump in someone's life, not a life-changing tragedy.

Robots among us

There are many examples now how robots could play a role in medicine and generally in people's everyday lives.

Telenoid R1, designed by the Osaka University and Advanced Telecommunications Research Institute International, is a teleoperated android robot developed to transmit an individual's presence. It appears and behaves as a minimalistic persona, allowing viewers to feel as if an acquaintance far away is next to them. A remote presence might be a grandchild for the elderly with whom they can communicate in a natural setting. Another potential companion, Actroid, also developed by Osaka University, is a type of humanoid robot that has a visually strong human-likeness modeled on an average young woman of Japanese descent. It can mimic such lifelike functions as blinking, and breathing, and is able to recognize speech and respond in kind.

The Vasteras Giraff is a mobile communication tool similar to Skype that enables the elderly to communicate with the outside world. It is remote controlled and has wheels, a camera, and a monitor. The Aethon TUG is an automated system that travels through hospital corridors and moves medication, linens, food, and supplies from one space to another. It even navigates elevators. New models serving quite different purposes come out almost every month now.

Trend 7. Surgical and Humanoid Robots

Atlas is 1.83 m tall, weighs 150 kg, is made of graded aluminum and titanium, can walk on rough terrain, withstand being hit by projectiles, and balance on one leg. It costs about $2 million. It is a bipedal humanoid that Boston Dynamics presented during a 2013 conference. Inspired by the 2011 Fukushima Daiichi nuclear disaster, six different teams will compete in the 2014 DARPA Robotics Challenge to test the robot's ability to perform tasks such as including getting in and out of a vehicle, driving it, opening a door, and using a power tool. In the near future its sensate hands will enable Atlas to use tools designed for human use. By having cameras and intelligent software it can perform environment–dependent tasks such as identifying the piece of wood it was told to pick up and then stooping down to grab it.

Nine customers took a seat at "Robots Bar and Lounge" in Ilmenau, East Germany while a humanoid robot called Carl measured out spirits into cocktail shakers and engaged them in limited conversations. The robot was built by mechatronics engineer Ben Schaefer at H&S–Robots. He has spent 23 years in the field using parts of disused industrial robots from the German firm KUKA.

A robot companion developed by H&S–Robots.

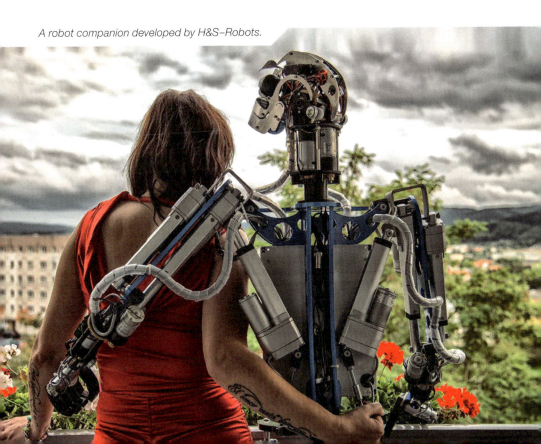

Trend 7. Surgical and Humanoid Robots

Veebot, a California-based start-up, combined robotics with image-analysis software to draw blood from patients safely. The machine restricts the patient's blood flow, an infrared light shines on the skin, and a camera searches for a vein. Then it checks the vein via ultrasound to make sure it is on target. In less than one minute, it draws blood. Its success rate is about 83 percent, the same as humans. They are aiming at 90 percent before moving to clinical trials.

A company based in Israel, Given Imaging, developed the first pill cameras that can be swallowed and send information to a receiver outside the body. Several research groups are working on making these capsules self-maneuvering. A European collaboration of researchers called ARES is currently testing a way for multiple capsules to automatically snap together. It means capsules could be assembled into a more complex device once safely in the stomach after each is swallowed individually. Such capsules could perform a different task such as imaging, providing power, or taking samples. Inside the stomach the capsules would link together to create a snake-like device that slithers through the intestines, performing tasks that are more complex than those that can be performed by a single capsule or several free-floating ones.

In the distant future, medical drones could deliver supplies and drugs to conventionally unreachable areas. For example, 85% of roads are inaccessible during the wet season in sub-Saharan Africa, cutting off the population, and hindering transportation of medical supplies. The list of examples could go on almost without end.

Medical robotics is still a young, unexplored field made possible by technical improvements over the past couple decades, meaning that the potential benefits provided by such robots are not fully understood. They have only gone through a few generations, one can make although educated guesses about the influence of robots on medicine in the near future such as better medical outcomes, tissue engineering, gene therapy, and rapid interventions.

A fundamental challenge with automated robotic surgery is decision-making. Like surgeons now, a robot has to be able to spot a vein, know to avoid it, and to detect if it starts bleeding. Guang-Zhong Yang at Imperial College London thinks that aiming for fully autonomous surgical robots is not the right approach. Due to the fact that people are pretty good in terms of decision-making and learning; while robots are good at doing precise movements, a combination of both could be the solution.

In support of this notion the National Robotics Initiative is already underway- "co-robots acting in direct support of and in a symbiotic relationship with human partners." The question here is whether we will be able to control robots without untoward consequences. The famous science fiction writer Isaac Asimov anticipated the need for basic rules when he formulated his Three Laws of Robotics in his 1942 story "Runaround."

1. A robot may not injure a human being or, through inaction, allow a human being to come to harm.
2. A robot must obey the orders given to it by human beings, except where such orders would conflict with the First Law.
3. A robot must protect its own existence as long as such protection does not conflict with the First or Second Law.

Much later Asimov added a "zeroth" law that said "a robot may not harm humanity, or, by inaction, allow humanity to come to harm."

The paper that won an award at the 2014 IEEE International Conference on Human–Robot Interaction described robots communicating with people by human-like body language, gestures and cues. The authors think this is a crucial step to placing robots in homes where they might have a better, more natural interaction with people. Such efforts are needed to close the gap between people and the robots they create.

Score of availability: 5
Focus of attention: Medical professionals
Websites & other online resources: The Society of Robotic Surgery (http://www.srobotics.org/), Medical Robots News by IEEE (http://spectrum.ieee.org/robotics/medical-robots)
Companies & start-ups: H&S Robots (http://www.hs-robots.de), Boston Dynamics (http://www.bostondynamics.com/), da Vinci Surgery (http://www.davincisurgery.com/)
Books: I, Robot by Asimov
Movies: Prometheus (2012), Ender's Game (2013)

Trend 8. Genomics and Truly Personalized Medicine

I was about to become a medical student when the completion of the Human Genome Project was announced. The genetic information of a person's DNA was finally made available. I remember being thrilled at the opportunities that advances of genomics could provide humanity with. When I was working on my PhD, the Personal Genome Project garnered worldwide attention by aiming to sequence and publicize the complete genomes and share the medical records of 100,000 volunteers. Since the completion of the Human Genome Project in 2003, we have envisioned an era of personalized medicine in which everyone receives customized therapy and personalized dosages.

According to the Personalized Medicine Coalition (PMC) there are so far only about 150 cases in which personal genomics can be applied. These are based on evidence. As we move forward, we will increasingly have opportunities to use DNA analysis at the patient's bedside. This should be an obligatory step before actually prescribing any medications. Doing so means that patients would get a drug and dosage exactly customized to their unique genomic, thus metabolic background. Fast, accurate, and widely available DNA sequencing will be needed to reach this goal.

During my PhD thesis defense I was fortunate to have on my board of opponents Joel Dudley, PhD, Assistant Professor of Genetics and Genomic Sciences and Director of Biomedical Informatics at Mount Sinai School of Medicine. He and his team in New York work on one of the most exciting projects in systems biology, bioinformatics, and genomics. When I asked him where he thought the field of genomics was heading, he openly talked about his own medical conditions and their relation to his genome.

"I think that one way that innovative technologies can help keep the human touch in medicine is by helping patients feel understood. One example is that I have Crohn's disease, which is an inflammatory bowel disease. I am pretty open about this when I give talks and then I show how having my whole genome sequenced helped me understand my disease and also helped me with choosing the right therapy. I have mutations in the TPMT gene that would suggest I would have increased side effects if I were to take 6–mercaptopurine, which is commonly prescribed for Crohn's disease. I think that human diseases are so complex and their manifestations in individuals are often so unique

that individuals affected by disease are often seeking to have the unique and personal characteristics of their disease understood."

He mentioned how he helped individuals with Crohn's disease better understand their condition by identifying mutations in their genome sequence that are likely affecting their disease either through modified drug response or different progression. He thinks that once a patient is given the DNA evidence proving that they are indeed challenged with a specific disease– and have a specific name of the parts of their genes that are broken– it can be comforting. It can also help them build stronger ties within a community of similarly affected individuals.

He sees parallels with the autism gene panels now offered at Mount Sinai. Autism is a puzzling disease with a strong genetic component, yet parents and affected individuals often have to fight misconceptions or overly simplistic models of the disease that are held by doctors and family members. Through Dr. Dudley's tests some of these individuals will find that they have specific genetic mutations linked to autism. Such hard biological evidence can be a tremendous relief to families because it can explain their daily struggles, and they can show this evidence to others.

Dr. Dudley has firm views about the challenges genomics face in its quest to becoming widely adopted. Current EMR systems do not fundamentally understand genomic information, and vendors are not motivated to solve this problem. One reason why physicians limit their engagement with genomic information is that they traditionally have not had much formal training in either genomics or its effect on developing diseases.

At Mount Sinai School of Medicine they developed the CLIPMERGE platform to help EMRs make intelligent use of genetic information in prescribing drugs. In oncology, which has a growing catalog of cancer–causing mutations, Foundation Medicine is offering targeted genomic tests to guide clinical decisions; unfortunately, it is necessary to sequence entire cancer genomes to do this.

Dr. Dudley's team uses state–of–the–art methods in genomics and systems biology to analyze specified networks of similar medical conditions while keeping traditional values in mind.

Trend 8. Genomics and Truly Personalized Medicine

"The problem with that is that we've forgotten what Greek physicians knew thousands of years ago, and that is the fact that the human body is a complex adaptive system with many connected dynamic components interacting and communicating on multiple levels—not only within the body, but also with the external environment. One hallmark of a complex adaptive system like the human body is that you cannot understand the whole by looking at individual parts and that the whole is always greater than the sum of the parts. In this light, the fact that medicine and biology are so siloed into domains or disease-focused specialties is, in my opinion, ridiculous, because that is not how it is in the human body. No disease manifests in isolation from the rest of an individual's physiology."

In the future, Dudley hopes it will be possible to define disease in terms similar to GPS coordinates. An individual's disease could be classified numerically in relation to other patients or diseases according to similarities with other patients or diseases. Partnerships with patients must be built where we can collect and analyze the streams of real-time information sent by consumer biosensors, and help predict when individuals are at increased risk. By prevention we shift our focus from disease treatment to maintaining human health and vitality.

Genome data for everyone

I envision a day when it will be quite common to have our genomes sequenced. The magic number will be 7 000 000 000 (global population) times 3 000 000 000 (number of base pairs in our DNA) equaling 2,1 * 1019 which is the number of base pairs that should soon be available. Based on trends in other industries such as mobile phones, I think the cost of sequencing a human genome will be close to zero, while the analysis needed to draw conclusions useful to medical decisions will be expensive.

Dr. Dudley agrees with me about the cost of sequencing, but he expects genome interpretation to eventually be free. Models will appear in which making huge investments in better genome interpretation tools or web services will be worthwhile because they will enable the collection of valuable information from a large population, capture attention, and somehow monetize that attention.

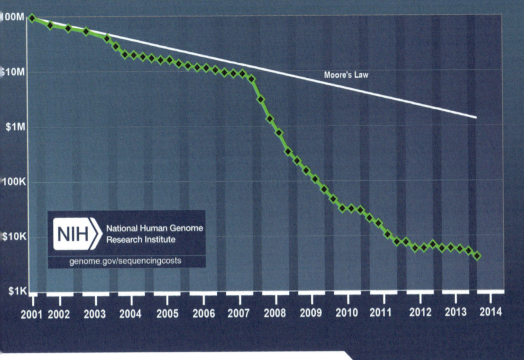

Typical cost of sequencing a human-sized genome over time on a logarithmic scale, as of 21 May 2014 estimated by the National Human Genome Research Institute.

Unfortunately, the broader clinical utility of genomics has not been firmly established yet. Examples exist in pharmacogenomics, covering the response given to particular drugs; and oncology where genomic information has strong scientific and clinical support for informing clinical decisions. But without established clinical usefulness backed by evidence, third-party payers will not be amenable to reimbursing the costs of applying genomics technologies.

In 2009 I was invited to the Science Foo Camp at the headquarters of Google, called Googleplex. There I met Professor George Church, world-famous Harvard professor of Genetics. I asked for his thoughts on the future of genome sequencing, and he scheduled a long call so we could discuss this, and the mission of this book, at length.

Trend 8. Genomics and Truly Personalized Medicine

"The human touch is there, it has worked for long, sitting by the patient's bedside and trying to lift their spirits. Although with the advances of human genomics, parts of the process have become automated, medical professionals cannot practice the way they used to, it is no longer the same human contact that we had before. Patients usually get interested in new technologies first; therefore there is a constant request that physicians start using them. Medical professionals don't have to get detailed training about how magnetic resonance imaging works, they just need to know why it works."

Thousands of things can be done in genetics. But its real promises have not yet arrived. Professor Church explained that educating the general public and medical professionals is the biggest next step. With preventive medicine, people could be proactive in taking care of their own health rather than being reactive as we are now.

He questioned the quality of data obtained and used in genomics, though he was optimistic in envisioning portable DNA sequencing with smartphones; new kinds of eyeglasses that can see allergens and pathogens in the environment, and thereby change the way we work, go to school, or live our lives. The first GPS devices were hard to use and too complicated. But as the industry improved, instructions became simple enough for people to navigate smoothly. The same scenario can be expected in genomics. What is needed though, according to Professor Church, is better software.

Genomics can change lives

I have had genomic tests identifying some of the mutations I carry as well as partially sequencing my genome with three companies. Navigenics, Pathway Genomics, and Gentle provided me with a thorough analysis and a huge text file that contains my genomic information. It gave me a clear picture about how such services operate, and I probably experienced what other consumers went through. I simply opened the company's website, ordered my test, received a sampling tube a week later, and provided saliva sample. Certain companies require customers to provide almost 10 ml of saliva, a challenging process that can take half an hour. I sent the sample tube back and was notified of the results by e-mail.

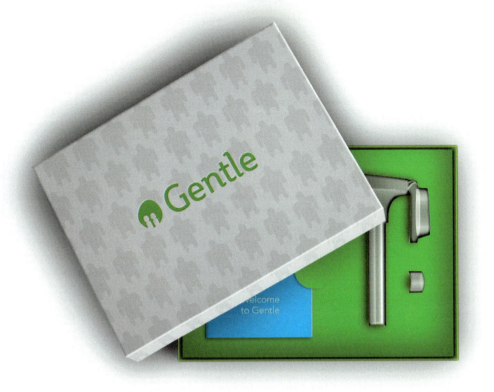

The sampling kit from Gentle.

With a few exceptions such as carrier status for rare conditions or certain pharmacogenomic features (meaning what drugs I am sensitive to), the information provided was not useful. Certainly it did not influence any of my medical decisions, except Gentle that provided definite answers to my questions. Accordingly, I was not surprised that the FDA warned the Google-backed company 23andMe to stop performing what it regarded as a medical test without its approval, and without physician oversight. The service had to change the way it analyzed and released consumers' genomic data. Given constant improvements, the service should become better and better over by time.

Recent news reports highlight the growing importance of genomics. Anne Morriss gave birth to a boy with a rare genetic disease, MCAD deficiency, which affects fat metabolism. It turned out that her sperm bank donor carried a rare genetic mutation for it just like she did. The unfortunate experience led her to launch a new company, Genepeeks, with a scientist at Princeton University. It takes the DNA of sperm donors and recipients and creates "virtual babies"

Trend 8. Genomics and Truly Personalized Medicine

or in–silica offsprings that can be screened for genetic diseases. They hope to make the technology available to any couple trying to conceive.

For about 25 years, it has been known that traces of fetal DNA can be detected in a pregnant woman's blood. A study in The New England Journal of Medicine recently demonstrated how DNA sequencing can detect an extra copy of a chromosome with remarkable accuracy, heralding perhaps a new era in prenatal DNA testing. Out of 1,914 young, healthy pregnant women, just eight fetuses had an extra chromosome. The test detected them all. What if in the future we could predict all diseases, main features of a child and even complex traits the live offspring will have to deal with? Would it lead to a genetic discrimination before birth?

I called Edward Abrahams to discuss such issues and the future of genomics. He is the President of the PMC launched in 2004 to educate the public and policy makers. It aims to promote new ways of thinking about healthcare, and represents over 225 innovators, academic, industry, patient, provider, and payer communities. In the 3rd edition of "The Case for Personalized Medicine", the PMC described a bright future involving genomics and big data:

"Imagine a physician sitting down with his laptop and a morning cup of coffee. On a website that he uses to help manage his practice, an alert pops up. It tells him that a series of studies have demonstrated a connection between multiple rare mutations found in 10 percent of people and the likelihood that they might convert to type 2 diabetes. Nearly all of his patients have had their entire genome sequenced and entered into their electronic medical record – a process that takes only a week, costs a few hundred dollars, and is reimbursed by insurance companies because of the many benefits it provides to lifelong health management.
He conducts a quick search of his 2,000 patient database and finds about 80 who are at risk. To half of those patients, he sends a strong reminder and advice on diet and lifestyle choices they can take to avoid the disease. To the other half, whose medical records reveal pre–diabetic symptoms; he sets up appointments to consider more proactive treatment with drugs that can prevent the onset of disease."

Trend 8. Genomics and Truly Personalized Medicine

Abrahams told me that after the Human Genome Project was completed expectations were unrealistic. This often happens with technological breakthroughs. But over time that breakthrough is likely to transform the practice of medicine. It takes a long time to change regulatory patterns, and everything that needs to be addressed, but that is what PMC was created to do. Unfortunately, progress has been only incremental in taking products using genomic information to the market.

He believes that more evidence is needed showing that targeted therapies and personalized medicine can not only improve patient outcomes, but also save money when incorporated into the health system over the long term. If researchers can show that this is true, then they will have a much better argument to make to payers.

PMC's hope is that a more efficient system will appear by targeting therapies and thus avoiding inefficient side effects. A second purpose of the PMC is education given that most of the public and many providers do not really understand what this is really about. The PMC hopes that when people do understand how it works, both stakeholders can benefit. Sequencing costs will drop to zero. In twenty years we will stop talking about personalized medicine as it will no longer be anything special.

Oxford Nanopore, a UK-based company, released its MinION sequencer in 2013. It can read short DNA fragments, exists on a USB drive sized device, and can perform the actual sequencing on a laptop. Although it fell short of its originally high expectations, the device is proof of concept that we can bring genomic sequencing to the masses.

QuantuMDx, a new player on the market that lets any laypeople run DNA analyses, tried to crowdfund its development on Indiegogo. Its founders envisioned a handheld DNA laboratory device in every bathroom cabinet for at-home testing for ailments such as flu.

Showcasing how genomics could transform society, researchers at Penn State and the Catholic University of Leuven developed a statistical model for mapping facial features using racial, gender, and genetic markers. Now it is almost possible to create accurate mugshots using only DNA. Envision a crimeless world in which whoever leaves DNA behind can be traced easily in seconds.

It should not be surprising that Craig Venter, one of the fathers of modern genomics, described a really interesting method in his recent book, Life at the Speed of Light. He claimed to have built a prototype of a "Digital Biological Converter" that would allow biological teleportation.

Trend 8. Genomics and Truly Personalized Medicine

One could receive DNA sequences over the Internet and synthesize proteins, viruses, and even living cells meaning the teleportation of life. The prototype can only produce DNA currently, not proteins or living cells. But given the history of Venter's previous ventures one can expect it to advance soon. It could not only teleport vaccines, antibiotics or insulin to long distances, but even provide patients with personalized drugs right away. This is the quest personalized medicine has to take on by using more and more advanced genomic analyses. Our blueprint, known as the DNA, is heavily responsible for making us different individuals; therefore it should start playing a much bigger role in making diagnoses and prescribing customized treatments in the near future.

Score of availability: 6
Focus of attention: Researchers and patients
Websites & other online resources: The Personalized Medicine Coalition (http://www.personalizedmedicinecoalition.org/), GenomeWeb (http://www.genomeweb.com/), PHG Foundation (http://www.phgfoundation.org/)
Companies & start–ups: Oxford NanoPore (https://www.nanoporetech.com), Gentle (https://gentlelabs.com/)
Books: Exploring Personal Genomics by Dudley & Karczewski
Movies: Gattaca (1997), Splice (2009)

Trend 9. Body Sensors Inside and Out

What do we do when we need to measure different health parameters? We go to a lab and provide blood sample; or to the hospital where they measure blood pressure, ECG, and perform other diagnostic tests. After that we wait and bring the results to the doctor to discuss the next step. If we need a radiology imaging or a laboratory test, it might take a lot of time due to waiting lists worldwide. When I wanted to get my DNA sequenced I provided saliva sample and sent it to direct–to–consumer genomic companies that gave me online access to the results a few weeks later. They even provided a genetic counselor to interpret the data for me over the phone.

There are only a few medical parameters that people have been able to measure at home by themselves. Blood pressure and blood glucose levels are prime examples. We rely on healthcare institutions to obtain data about our own body. But for how long?

What if medical professionals focused on solving this shortcoming instead of spending time and energy on obtaining whatever data is required for solving a medical problem? What if blood tests, biomarkers, imaging, or simply blood pressure values were available right away?

This notion has driven the development of newer kinds of sensors that can be embedded, implanted, or worn in order to measure health parameters in a way that hasn't been accessible before. Fitness and sport have been two areas that have put the most pressure on developers to come up with sensors that can ease, gamify, and improve an individual's health.

A massively increasing number of gadgets, solutions, and technologies now make such measurements possible, convenient, and simple. It will be a challenge to find a balance between using an increasing amount of personal tech and only that we actually need. During one of my talks I took an ECG with my smartphone using FDA–approved AliveCor. Afterwards a colleague told me that his wife would do an ECG on herself every 5 minutes if she had the device. Overuse is normal during the hype phase.

Downloads of smartphone medical apps declined after their initial release. In this spirit I remain confident we will find a proper balance for a technology's use over time. Wearing hundreds of health trackers should not be the solution even though insightful trackers add value to our lives. The best scenario might be to include tiny sensors in clothing and accessories–contact lenses or rings–making the measurement of health data elegant and invisible

Trend 9. Body Sensors Inside and Out

compared to a Holter ECG monitor that is worn for 24 hours.

According to Nielsen's 2013 Connected Life Report 15% of consumers who know the term "wearable" are wearing one. Of those who owned such a device, 61% owned fitness wristbands and 45% owned smartwatches. Costs per person need to go down to encourage mass adoption of these devices, which is exactly where the industry is heading.

In 2013, 96% of all connected wearable devices were activity trackers, 3% were smartwatches, and 1% were smart glasses. Tellingly, 82% of users believe that wearable tech has enhanced their lives. By 2017, 64 million shipments of such devices are expected (8 times larger than in 2012). Global spending on wearable technology is estimated to be $19 billion by 2018.

PSFK, a content network, released "The Future of Wearable Tech," which identified several possible inventions that let users feel one another from afar. A smart ring might let us feel a user far away; earbuds might monitor a wearer's mood and select the next song to match it. Zoomable contact lenses could assist patients with degenerative retinal disorders; low–voltage electronic make–up could activate gadgets by predetermined facial expressions; and ingestible password pills developed by Motorola and Proteus Health could let us log into websites or devices only by being in the proximity of the device.

Sensors can be embedded in tissue (pacemaker), ingestible (smart pills), epidermal (smart skin or digital tattoo), wearable (clothing or jewelry), and external (traditional blood pressure monitors and smartwatches). As their number is increasing quickly, 2014 might be a turning point when health wearables become mainstream and most people acknowledge the advantages this range of gadgets might offer.

Wearing invisible sensors

Given that wearable sensors will influence daily life, they have to be tiny, practically invisible, and yet technically accurate. Once I watched a presentation by Professor Takao Someya, PhD, of The University of Tokyo. He is the Project Director of Someya's Bio–Harmonized Project. His team has been working on the first flexible wireless sensor that can function as electrical Band–Aids or diapers.

His goal is to develop electronic devices that interface with living bodies, taking advantage of features of organic molecules. Such devices can be fabricated using biocompatible inks, creating circuits with millions of soft biosensors that can safely communicate with biological tissue.

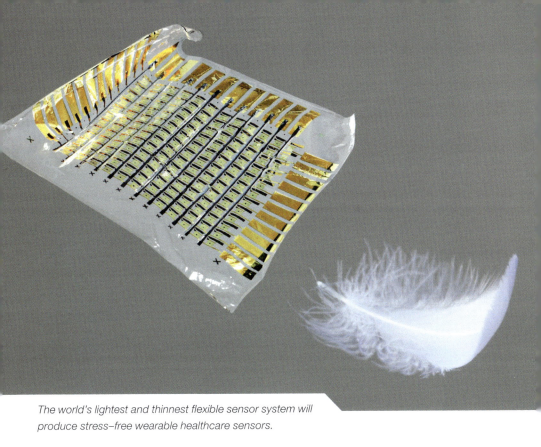

The world's lightest and thinnest flexible sensor system will produce stress-free wearable healthcare sensors.

When rigid materials are implanted into biological tissue they cause inflammation. This barrier hinders embedding sensors such as blood glucose detectors for long periods. In order to overcome this, Someya's team has focused on biocompatible organic semiconductors as opposed to conventional inorganic materials such as silicon. Potential developments include smart catheters, wheelchairs, and flexible health sensors that can constantly monitor certain parameters.

Professor Someya described the goal of his research:

"These probes will be able to sense the electrical and chemical signals of the billions of neurons which exist inside the human brain, and will enable high-resolution visualization of real-time neuron activities. By utilizing novel organic bio-devices, we aim to complete a visualization of complicated neural networks, and subsequently, a visualization of the activities of a whole brain that is an aggregation of billions of neurons."

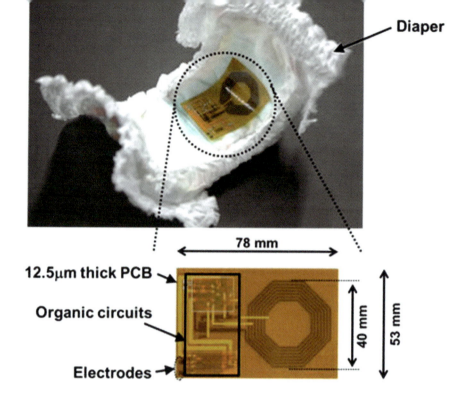

The world's first soft wireless organic sensor system detects liquid and wirelessly transmits data. The sensor is powered wirelessly and can be mounted to diapers or Band–Aids for disposable use.

Imagine that such sensors in the body and implanted in everyday devices could revolutionize the way we collect information about our health. Measuring easily quantifiable data is the gateway to better health. The future belongs to digestible, embedded, and wearable sensors. The latter works like a thin e-skin. These sensors will measure vital signs and important health parameters 24 hours a day, transmitting data to the cloud and sending alerts to medical systems, for example, when a stroke is happening real time. It will call the ambulance and transmit pertinent data.

One can swallow digital sensors that gather and store data to an external device. In gastrointestinal diseases, for example, swallowing a device that included a video camera could render an instant diagnosis by combining lab results with colonoscopy pictures.

Recently, Equivital provided the Oxford Kidney Unit with data to support the development of a tool that would prevent adverse events in patients with kidney failure who were undergoing haemodialysis (a method

Trend 9. Body Sensors Inside and Out

used to remove waste products such as creatinine, urea and free water from the blood). Equivital developed a sensor that continuously monitors vital signs including pulse oximetry, oxygen saturation, and core temperature. These are known risk factors for adverse events of dialysis. The company develops other applications for medical, pharmaceutical, and military use as well.

A thin sensor wore like a digital tattoo measuring health parameters.

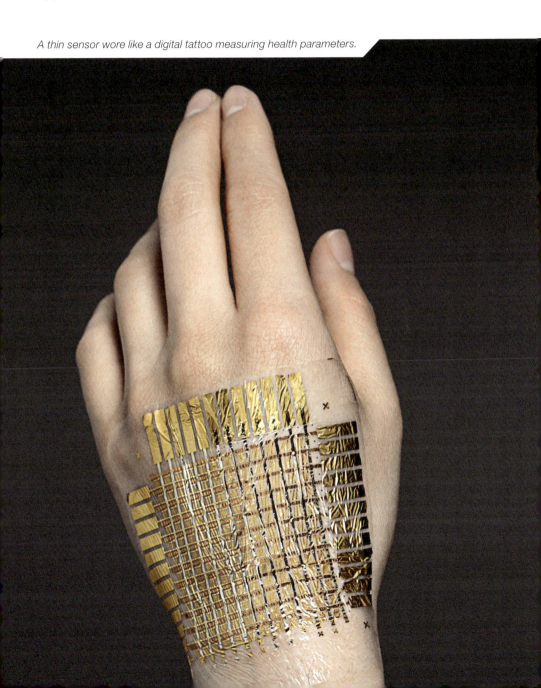

Trend 9. Body Sensors Inside and Out

MC10, based in Cambridge Massachusetts, has developed a platform that combines conventional electronics with novel mechanics. It enables a new generation of thin electronic systems for sports, fitness, cosmetics, healthcare, energy and defense. They demonstrated their first product at the CES conference. It featured skullcap electronics to measure the impact force an athlete sustains during contact sports. It thus suggests whether or not players have received a potentially dangerous blow to the head. The company tirelessly develops silicon devices thinned to a fraction of the width of a human hair, uses stretchable metallic interconnects, and elastic rubberlike polymers to form complete powered systems that sense, measure, analyze, and communicate information.

A Japanese mobile carrier and materials developer Toray announced a joint project Hitoe (Japanese for "one layer"), a cloth containing nanofibers coated in a transmittable layer. Using electrodes, the clot can measure pulse and even metrics resembling a cardiogram with the plan to transmit the data to the smartphone of the owner of the smart cloth. This was considered one of the first steps in designing a new kind of clothing.

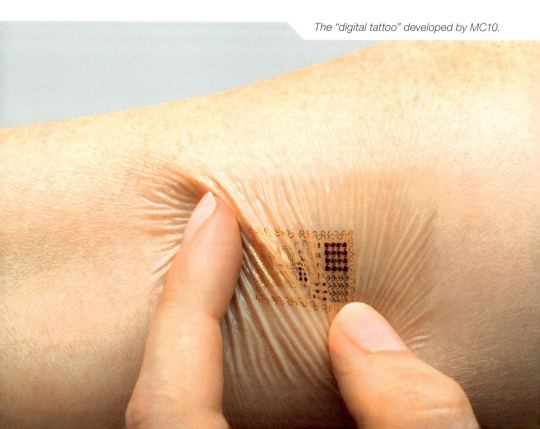

The "digital tattoo" developed by MC10.

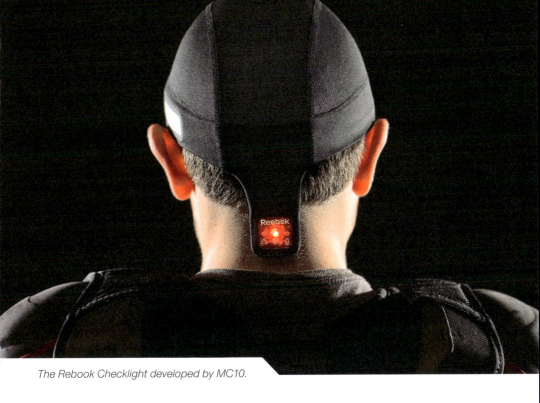

The Rebook Checklight developed by MC10.

Designer Kerri Wallace recently created a shirt that responds to body heat, and what mood that person is in. Workout gear developed by Radiate Athletics reports visual activity levels of the wearer in real-time. The company ithlete aims to tell users when to train more, and when to rest based continual heart rate monitoring.

HexoSkin has developed the first electronic shirt that tracks movement, respiration, and pulse. Users such as professional athletes, astronauts, and sport enthusiasts put the shirt on, plug in the device, and see their body metrics displayed on a smartphone right away. These statistics are uploaded to the user's online account and generate detailed recommendations on training and general health. Feedback on physical activity, stress, sleep quality, nocturnal breathing, and heart rate are all expensive at the moment, but a decline is expected in coming years.

The smart bra has successfully been tested in over 500 patients to date. It shows a 74% correlation to actual cancer stages in all types of breast tissue. Smart shoes connected to a smartphone guide the user to where he wants to get. Be prepared when famous fashion designers start to focus on such innovations.

Trend 9. Body Sensors Inside and Out

Constantly monitoring our health?

Scanadu, founded in 2011 and based at the NASA Ames Research Center in Mountain View, California, finished a successful crowdfunding campaign that raised $1.66 million from 8,800 backers to develop medical technology devices for consumers. The prototype of the first product, the Scanadu Scout, is a portable device that measures parameters such as temperature, heart rate, blood oxygenation, respiratory rate, ECG, and blood pressure. It was shipped to backers in March, 2014, and the company plans to make the device available for consumers in the first quarter of 2015.

A rival Wi-Fi enabled sensor developed at National Taiwan University can be embedded in a tooth cavity and measure jaw movements, drinking, chewing, coughing, speaking and even smoking. The results are wirelessly transmitted. If the sensor receives all the appropriate inputs it can potentially curb assorted addictions, from smoking to drinking alcohol excessively.

A company called iHealth Lab is working on an ambulatory blood pressure monitor, wireless ambulatory ECG, and a wearable pulse oximeter that could be used in ambulances. Kolibree has developed a smart toothbrush that monitors brushing habits and helps users improve their dental health. A vitamin-sized ingestible pill camera Is PillCamSB weighing less than 4 grams was approved for human use by the FDA. It can monitor pressure, pH, temperature, gastrointestinal motility, and detect ulcers, early signs of tumors, and bleeding within the small bowel. Sensors for almost any health parameter and any body part are becoming available. The developments described above have hit the market only in the last one to two years.

In addition to digestible and wearable sensors, imagine similar wireless technology providing real-time data from an artificial pancreas or recording brain waves constantly. Medtronic is a company a thirty-year history of innovation in diabetes technology. It brought the first insulin pump to market in 1983. In 2013, the FDA approved their fully automated "artificial pancreas," a device that closely mimics the insulin delivery of a working pancreas by continuously monitoring glucose levels and adjusting insulin delivery, all with little or no patient interaction.

Retinal implants that restore sight are already on the market. Second Sight makes an implant that includes a video camera and transmitter in a pair of glasses. Video images are converted into a series of electrical pulses transmitted wirelessly to an array of electrodes laying on the surface of the

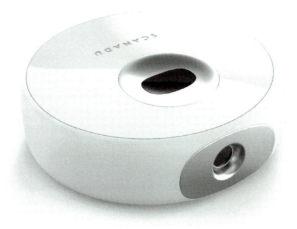

The Scanadu Scout.

retina. The pulses stimulate the retina's remaining healthy cells, which relay them to the optic nerve.

Transparent 1–micron thick circuits embedded in a polymer membrane can be used in contact lenses to monitor the buildup of pressure in the eye for those with glaucoma, or continuously measure blood glucose levels in tears for diabetics. The technology is getting closer to making 24/7 monitoring a reality and matter of choice for patients. A skin patch dispenses drugs continuously and can determine when to stop. It can release therapeutic agents based on a patient's body temperature. Such patches could become entirely wireless and brought to the market in less than five years.

Wearable devices could use biometrics besides facial structures, expressions, DNA, or iris patterns. A Canadian start–up, Bionym, has developed biometric identification using the unique patterns of a user's ECG, which varies according to the size, shape, and position of the heart in one's body.

Leslie Saxon from the University of Southern California's Keck School of Medicine addressed the possibility of wearing more and more sensors in and on our body. A baby born five or ten years from now could be tattooed with an integrated circuit at birth that could monitor ECG, physical activity, nutritional status, sleep duration, breathing rate, body temperature, and hydration, all generating a huge amount of data that can be used in health management, disease prediction, and even monetization for large healthcare companies. The data could be transmitted to smartphones or tablets. Applications would give parents and pediatricians insights into the baby's health and condition in real–time. The same scenario is available for adults, especially soldiers or athletes. She warned, however, that we must be cautious. The point is "using

Trend 9. Body Sensors Inside and Out

machines to amplify their humanity, not to scare the heck out of them".

Daniel Reed, a frequent government advisor on science and technology policy, addressed the growing importance of wearables in 2013. He said that even though everyone is different, today's medical treatments are still quite generic. In a few years, we may have wearable and perhaps implantable metabolic diagnostics constituting an early health warning system.

Max Knoblauch, a reporter of Mashable.com, was not persuaded by the wearable revolution and Quantified Self movement. He therefore measured numerous daily parameters for 30 days, which he called the most miserable, self-aware 30 days he has ever spent. He used MyFitnessPal to track running, Sleepbot to track sleeping habits, and Fitbit to measure his physical activity. Some results were obvious while a few things were a surprise such as having a normal sleeping schedule. He learned that while the wearable revolution is here, we still have to wait for the right gadgets to appear that combine the many existing trackers into one. As if to underscore this, a recent study concluded that one-third of wearable device owners a stopped using them within six months.

Dr. Kamal Jethwani from the Center for Connected Health in Boston believes that the goal should not be to make people wear a activity tracker for a whole year, but to wear it when it is meaningful. There will be unintended consequences in the future with wearable devices, but this future can be human centric if we, at the level of the whole society, focus on the real potentials and risks. This is a discussion we all have to initiate now.

Score of availability: 5
Focus of attention: Patients
Websites & other online resources: Crunchwear (http://www.crunchwear.com/)
Companies & start-ups: MC10 (http://www.mc10inc.com/), Equivital (http://www.equivital.co.uk/), Scanadu (https://www.scanadu.com/)
Books: Sensor Technologies: Healthcare, Wellness and Environmental Applications by McGrath & Scanaill
Movies: Minority Report (2002), The Avengers (2012)

Trend 10. The Medical Tricorder and Portable Diagnostics

There was an imaginary device called the medical tricorder on the 1960s television show "Star Trek." Used by Dr. Leonard McCoy, it instantly diagnosed an infinite number of medical conditions. A detachable, high-resolution, hand-held scanner sends life-sign information to the tricorder itself, which can check all organ functions and detect the presence of dangerous organisms. An additional feature not relevant to the mission of this book is its data banks on non-human species that make it possible to treat other life-forms as well.

For decades the tricorder has been an element of science fiction, but it seemed it might be reality soon when the Qualcomm Tricorder X Prize was announced in 2012, promising to award $10 million to the first team to build a medical tricorder. Over 230 teams from 30 countries entered the competition. The prize guidelines require that the device should diagnose 15 different medical conditions ranging from sore throat, sleep apnea, to colon cancer across 30 people in 3 days through a consumer friendly interface.

Nowadays, we are getting closer to the tricorder becoming an everyday item. As our smartphones become increasingly small, handheld medical laboratories it seems we do not have to look much further. With over one billion smartphones and 3 billion mobile phones worldwide, they have begun to play an important role in determining how we communicate, shop, or find new contacts. Almost all medical issues have a relevant smartphone application, and the number is still growing.

An estimated 500 million smartphone users, including medical professionals, consumers, and patients, will be using a healthcare-related application by 2015. Half of the more than 3.4 billion smartphone and tablet users will have downloaded mobile health applications by 2018.

The potential medical use of such smartphone applications and devices is clearly described by a story about Dr. Eric Topol, chief academic officer of Scripps Health, who was on a flight from Washington, DC to San Diego when the pilot asked whether there was a doctor on board. A passenger had severe chest pains. Topol put his iPhone into the AliveCor ECG bracket, performed an ECG and concluded that the patient was probably having a heart attack. An emergency landing followed and the patient survived.

According to Dr. Topol, the smartphone will be the hub of the future of medicine serving as a health-medical dashboard. He is famous for saying that

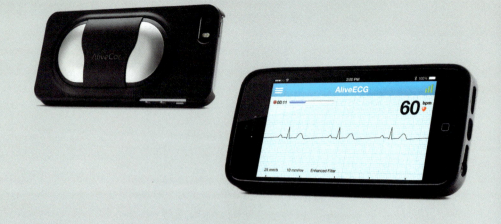

AliveCor from front and back views.

these days he prescribes a lot more applications than medications to his patients.

The founder and Chief Medical Officer of the company behind AliveCor is Dr. David E. Albert whom I met at the NASA Research Park in Moffett Field, California in 2013. Since then, I have been teaching medical students to use AliveCor and other portable devices in practice. Dr. Albert told me the device has been used more than a dozen times in–flight to make diagnoses from myocardial infarction to atrial fibrillation.

"Many arrhythmias have been captured by patients. Atrioventricular Nodal Reentry Tachycardia (AVNRT) in a young man who had a Fontan procedure at birth is one example where two 2–week Holter studies did not find anything. Six months after carrying our device, the young man had AVNRT at 250 beats per minute and was converted with adenosine at an emergency room with a definitive diagnosis. Probably as important are all the episodes of non–arrhythmias which are confirmed by a physician remotely and enable the prevention of an expensive emergency room visit."

The product's global roll to many markets with the same type of professional services that they have in the US could be a next step. As proof, they recently announced the integration of ECG data into Practice Fusion. Further integration of such portable diagnostic devices into EMRs is expected soon.

Another example is the iBGStar, the first blood glucose meter that can be connected to the iPhone and iPod. It is supported by an iOS application and measures blood glucose levels simply by inserting a test strip into the device, which is connected to the iPhone or iPod.

Trend 10. The Medical Tricorder and Portable Diagnostics

Clinical laboratory and radiology at home

Complicated methods for identifying microbes or measuring biomarkers have been the domain of laboratories equipped with expensive machines. Now this is moving to our homes. Biomeme designed a small, low–cost device that allows smartphone users with minimal laboratory skills to detect numerous diseases by replicating DNA. This is now only available in laboratories worldwide through expensive qPCR (quantitative polymerase chain reaction) machines that can amplify and quantify a DNA molecule.

An "optical lab on a chip" developed by researchers at UCLA measures 170,000 different molecules from cancer markers to insulin levels by using changes in light intensity. Only 7.5 cm high and weighing 60 grams, the device is able to detect viruses and single layer proteins down to 3 nanometers of size.

One of the largest European "lab on a chip" initiatives included thirteen partner institutions from eight countries. Its mission was to develop a portable laboratory that could deliver fast, low–cost, and reliable diagnostics. The project is called Labonfoil and received €5.3 billion in research funding from the European Union. The portable lab uses three 'smart cards' and a reader for analyzing the data, which can then be forwarded wirelessly to a computer, tablet, or smartphone.

With a few drops of blood, the first card can identify a specific protein whose presence is known to increase when cancer recurs. The second smart card can detect pathogens such as bacteria and viruses in food. The third card analyses phytoplankton concentrations in a sample of sea water.

A smart card of Labonfoil.

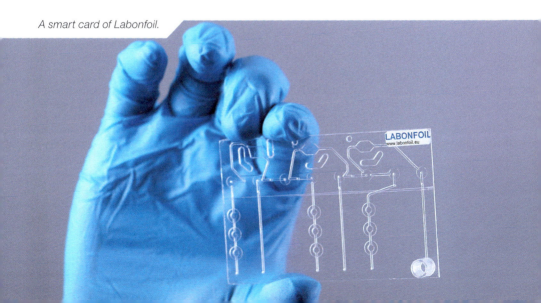

Northeastern University professor, Tania Konry, developed a small portable instrument called ScanDrop that can detect a variety of biological specimens. It contains a chip made of polymer or glass connected to equally tiny tubes. The extremely small-volume liquid sample such as water or biological fluid interacts with microscopic beads that in turn react with the lab test's search parameters including antibodies or cancer biomarkers.

If the device is clinically approved it might make it possible for lay people to carry out simple diagnostic procedures at home using their own smartphone. A smartphone application developed by University of Cambridge researchers turns a smartphone into a portable medical diagnostic device using colorimetric tests. After testing urine, saliva or other bodily fluid samples with a colorimetric test, the patient can take a photo of the test strip with the smartphone's camera and the Colorimetrix app analyzes the results by comparing them with pre-recorded calibration data.

Bringing radiology devices to patients' homes would likewise have clear benefits. About 60% of the world did not have access to ultrasound when the MobiUS SP1 was announced. It is an ultrasound device that can be used with a smartphone. Images are shared wirelessly, it has a storage capacity of 8GB, and it is portable and easy-to-use.

A cardiac intervention that uses MRI and CT machines to scan a patient's heart, create a model via 3D printing, and make a metallic mesh sleeve that can be implanted in the patient's chest was recently developed. This can be paired with a smartphone providing real-time and constant information about the heart and its health.

Evidence-based and customized Mobile Health

The number of medical mobile applications has been rising for years, although persuading users to keep using the apps is a challenge. The question is not whether such applications could be used in the practice of medicine or delivery of healthcare, but which ones and to what extent can be useful. Evidence based background is needed for implementing mobile apps in the clinical settings. In 2013, the FDA finally issued guidance that might facilitate the process, and encourages the development of mobile medical apps "that improve health care and provide consumers and health care professionals with valuable health information." Additionally, the FDA has a public health responsibility to ensure and oversee the safety and effectiveness of medical

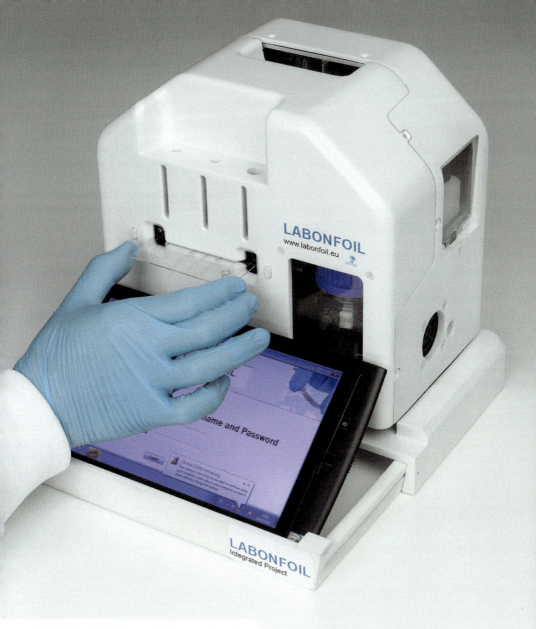

The Labonfoil device analyzing smart cards.

devices, which now include medical smartphone applications as well.

The first prescribed mobile application with health implications that is reimbursed by health insurance was launched in 2014. The Caterna Vision Therapy application is reimbursed by a German health insurance with 8.65 million Germans insured in partnership with a nationwide association of eye care centers. Since the 1st of April 2014, eye specialists have been prescribing it to patients.

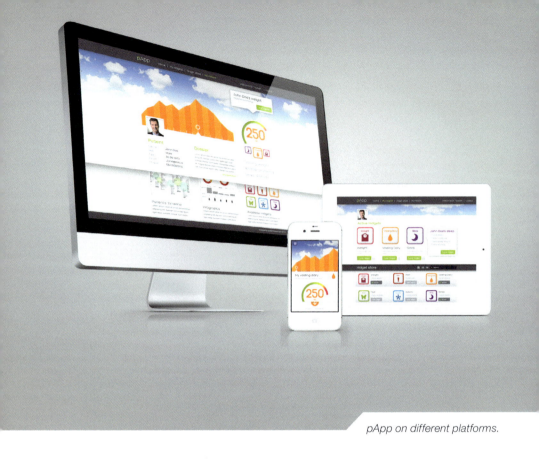

pApp on different platforms.

A growing problem is that patients and doctors find it harder and harder to choose the right app for their health management or work. Doing a search for a medical condition or specialty yields a long list of applications from which it is extremely hard to choose quality ones. Patients and caregivers can become better at that in the same way they learned to assess the quality of books, then websites. But it takes time. Regulation of medical apps that does not limit their capabilities would have benefits for all stakeholders.

Customized mobile apps such as the pApp could address this issue by letting doctors create mobile apps for their patients without knowing anything about mobile app development. They choose what functions (so–called bundles) the app should have, and the patient can download the app right away.

In the future as smartphones and tablets become common modalities, they will be equipped with display screens that can be rolled up like a scroll or folded like a wallet, making the devices easy to carry around. In–built projectors, seamless voice control, 3D screens, and holograms might represent the future of smartphones.

Trend 10. The Medical Tricorder and Portable Diagnostics

One possible direction might be the integration of health devices into smartphones instead of downloading apps on them. Apple introduced the iOS8 operating system and new devices that can measure basic health parameters. It is rumored that Apple is moving into the field of medicine with big announcements coming in 2014. These rumors mostly focus on a smartwatch that could monitor several health parameters from body temperature to pulse through a user interface that Apple usually designs. Similar to the case of the first iPhone, it could break the barriers for wider adoption of mobile health tracking.

There might be a time when clinical laboratories will vanish and be replaced by small, handheld, medically efficient devices that anyone can use without prior training. Measuring health and blood parameters could become a common and cheap process for even laypeople.

Score of availability: 7
Focus of attention: Patients and medical professionals
Websites & other online resources: Qualcomm Xprize (http://www.qualcommtricorderxprize.org/), iMedicalApps (http://www.imedicalapps.com/)
Companies & start-ups: Happtique (http://www.happtique.com/), AliceCor (http://www.alivecor.com/)
Books: The Next Web of 50 Billion Devices: Mobile Internet's Past, Present and Future by Ahmad
Movies: Star Trek (TV series)

Trend 11. Growing Organs in a Dish

In 2013, a survey of more than 2000 US adults by the Pew Research Center provided a picture of how people think about living much longer lives. Surprisingly, 60% of responders do not want to live past 90, and 30% do not want to live past 80. A slight majority said that if new medical treatments slowed the aging process and allowed the average person to live to at least 120; it would be "a bad thing for society". The more a person associates medical treatment with higher quality of life and the more one associates longevity with productivity, the more they favor life extension. The reason behind the survey results probably lies in the perception that aging is a devastating process and people cannot yet think clearly about the potentials of regenerative medicine to improve the quality of life.

When it becomes possible to grow new organs and replace old ones, rejuvenate the whole body or cure diseases with stem cell therapy, this perception is likely to dramatically change. Being able to help patients with chronic organ failure and solve the shortage of donor organs is something that scientists in regenerative medicine are all striving for. Regenerative medicine is an emerging field that has the potential to revolutionize several types of treatments from heart disease to neurodegenerative disorders; eradicate the organ donor shortage problem; and completely restore damaged tissues such as muscles, or tendons.

After watching Professor Anthony Atala's fascinating talk at TEDMED in 2009 about how his state-of-the-art lab grows human organs from muscles and blood vessels to bladders, I knew I had to talk with him to get the latest updates about this field. Professor Atala is the editor of several peer-reviewed journals and the leader of teams that focus on innovative topics from nanotechnology to growing human tissues. He is the Director of the Institute for Regenerative Medicine at Wake Forest Baptist Medical Center, has led US national professional and government committees, has ten clinical applications of technologies that were developed in his laboratory, has edited thirteen books, published more than 300 articles, applied for or received over 200 national and international patents; and is also a practicing surgeon. There is not enough room to list all his achievements.

He shared with me how he regards new treatments and technologies, and the patient-physician interaction:

Trend 11. Growing Organs in a Dish

"Obviously, our goal as physicians is to heal. But all physicians have been the position where everything available to us is still not enough to help the patient. I direct a team of more than 300 scientists working to develop new technologies – namely cell therapies and replacement tissues and organs – to fill some of this void. Many people say what we're doing sounds like science fiction. But all of these technologies are actually based on the body's innate ability to heal itself.

As "high-tech" as these treatments are, I do not believe they create distance between physicians and patients. Instead, they serve to deepen the bond. Being able to offer a patient a new treatment strengthens the physician-patient relationship. After all, hope of getting better is the reason they first put their trust in us."

He thinks a key to solving medical and scientific problems that seem futuristic now is the "need" as the driving force behind innovation that can lead to new treatments. Scientists and physicians should constantly ask themselves whether there is a better way to do this or how they can solve this problem.

The 3D printer at work on a kidney scaffold.

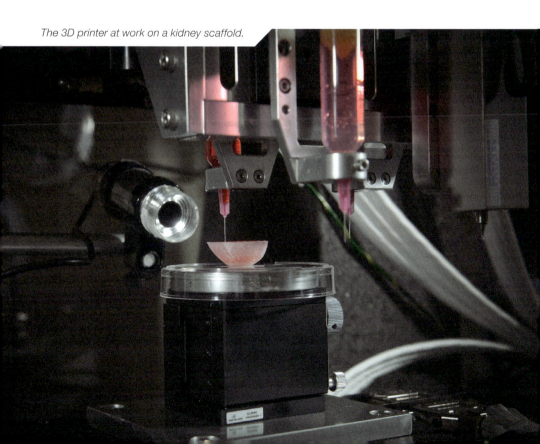

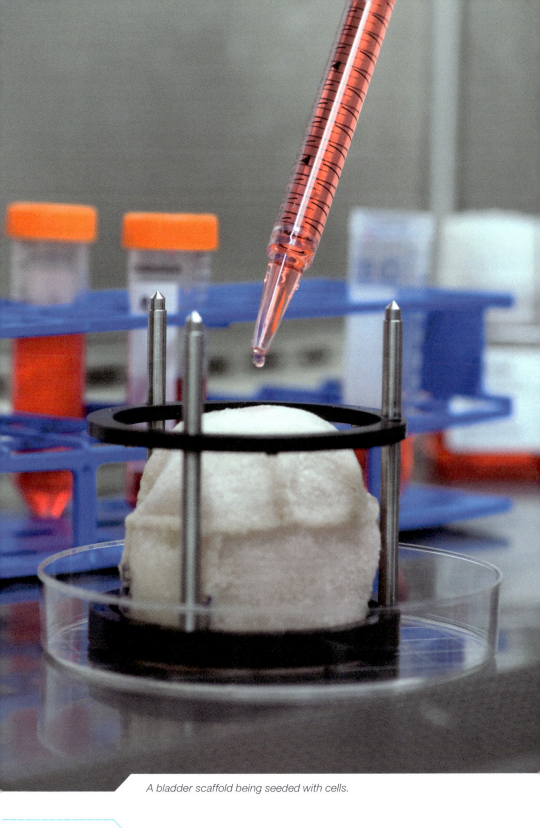
A bladder scaffold being seeded with cells.

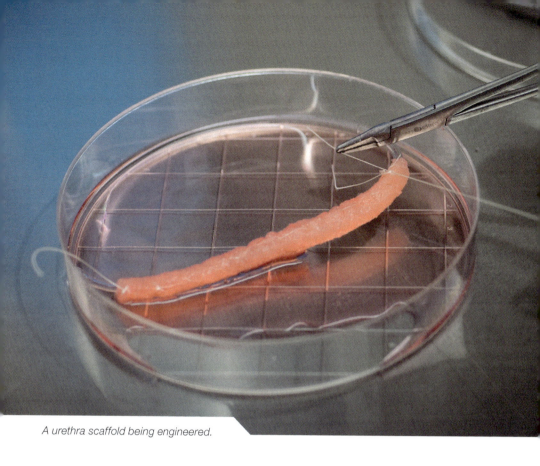

A urethra scaffold being engineered.

"Perseverance is also the key. If it does not work the first time, we need to try a different approach. Of course, there are many practical considerations involved in taking a new treatment from idea to reality, including the cost to develop and test new therapies, regulatory pathways and the ability to commercialize and make them widely available. But to me, the desire to solve problems and the drive to keep at it are at the heart of finding solutions."

Their goal at the institute is simply to develop new treatments to improve the lives of patients, although Professor Atala thinks it is best not to have pre-conceived notions about future directions, because that way they remain open to possibilities that their work uncovers. For example, maybe the entire kidney does not have to be replaced in patients with kidney failure. Researchers should not be wedded to that goal while ignoring other possibilities. Their focus is on the final goal of making the patient feel better, not on a particular way of making that happen.

Trend 11. Growing Organs in a Dish

As regenerative medicine is still a relatively new field of science, scientific progress alone will not drive the field forward. Manufacturing challenges and regulatory hurdles will also need to be successfully addressed.

In the 1980s Professor Robert Langer at MIT and surgeon Jay had the idea of combining 3D synthetic polymer scaffolds with cells in order to create new tissues and organs. While they were met with great skepticism

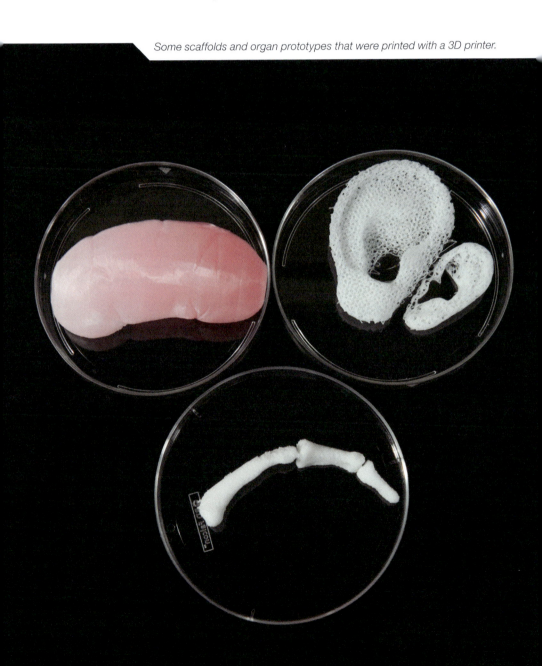

Some scaffolds and organ prototypes that were printed with a 3D printer.

and it was difficult to secure government funds, they managed to license the patents to companies, which provided them with funding for additional research. The idea has since become a cornerstone of tissue engineering and regenerative medicine, resulting in the creation of artificial skin for burn victims and, hopefully soon, whole organs. Professor Langer is known all over the world as a pioneer in the field of tissue engineering.

His research led to the invention of biodegradable polymer that could be placed inside a cancerous growth to deliver regular doses of medication to the target site, thus creating a safer and more effective process than typical chemotherapy. His three-dimensional polymer scaffolds have also been used by scientists to grow human cells in various configurations. A famous example is an ear grown in the lab.

At various stages of his scientific career he opted to face challenges that seemed impossible and about which the research community was skeptical. He and his team currently have many patents and FDA-approved products. When I asked him about the key for solving medical/scientific problems that seem too futuristic now, his response was direct and on the spot: "Believing that you can."

Total biocompatibility of implanted materials, the prevention of rejection by the host, and successful vascularization and innervation of implants are important areas to develop. There is work to be done.

The world of stem cells

Most adult stem cells are able to differentiate into only a limited number of specialized cell types, while embryonic stem cells (ESCs) are pluripotent meaning that such cells can differentiate into any cell types. The research around ESCs has bumped into ethical concerns as the derivation of ESCs requires the destruction of a blastocyst, an early-stage embryo that some people consider to be a viable form of life. Despite this, this area of science could make significant advances in the future years.

Stem cell research was revolutionized in 2006 when Dr. Shinya Yamanaka invented induced pluripotent stem cells ("iPS). These cells can then be rebooted to the so-called "stage zero" of life that is similar to their state after fertilization. Therefore, these stem cells are genetically reprogrammed to behave like embryonic stem cells and can be transformed into new tissues or organs. The first clinical trials are now using iPS cells to cure age-related

Trend 11. Growing Organs in a Dish

macular degeneration by reconstituting retinas and improving eyesight. If results are promising, it might soon be possible to be cured of Alzheimer's disease or cancer.

Researchers in Singapore developed a process whereby it is possible to derive adult stem cells from small samples of blood for stem cell reprogramming rather than using current invasive methods of obtaining bone marrow. Reprogrammed stem cells were transformed into human heart muscle cells that were even rhythmically beating.

Policy makers have substantial responsibility given that there are more and more stem cell clinics falsely claiming to offer safe and effective therapies for illnesses ranging from cardiovascular to Parkinson's disease.

In 2013, a University College London team made a new nose for a British man who lost his to cancer. Stem cells were obtained from the patient's fat tissue and grown in the lab for two weeks before being used to cover the nose scaffold. The new nose was implanted into the man's forearm so skin would grow over it. It is one of the several labs worldwide that are working on the futuristic idea of growing custom-made organs in the laboratory settings. So far, they have been able to make tear ducts, blood vessels, and windpipes, but researchers are optimistic that they can soon make more types of transplantable body parts. According to the team, it is like making a cake but using a different kind of oven.

University of Edinburgh researchers announced in 2014 that cells taken from humans were reprogrammed into stem cells and then grown into Type O red blood cells. It was the first time blood has been manufactured to appropriate quality and safety standards for transfusion into a human being. It might open the way to artificial blood soon.

In 2014 scientists succeeded in regenerating a living organ, the thymus, which produces immune cells. If the technique proves to be safe, it could pave the way for new therapies for people with damaged immune systems and genetic conditions affecting thymus development. Moreover, University of Cambridge researchers were able to identify ways to speed up the cellular processes by which human nerve cells mature. Functional nerve cells could be generated from skin cells and show the same functional characteristics as mature cells found in the body.

The ultimate goal is to grow new organs by printing them out in 3D in a fast, efficient, and safe way. A group named OxSyBio aims at developing 3D printing techniques to produce tissue-like synthetic materials for wound healing, drug delivery, organ repair and replacement. The technique they developed allows them to 3D print synthetic tissue–like materials from thousands of tiny water droplets each coated with a thin film mimicking a living cell's external membrane.

Although it seems most people do not want to live past 90 or 100 years, they will soon have to face that opportunity due to the rapid advances of regenerative medicine.

Score of availability: 3
Focus of attention: Researchers
Websites & other online resources: Centre for Regenerative Medicine (http://www.crm.ed.ac.uk/about/what–regenerative–medicine), Wake Forest Institute for Regenerative Medicine (http://www.wakehealth.edu/WFIRM/)
Companies & start–ups: Organovo (http://www.organovo.com/)
Books: Principles of Regenerative Medicine by Atala, Lanza, Thomson & Nerem; Regenerative Medicine Applications in Organ Transplantation by Orlando
Movies: Terra Incognita: The Perils and Promise of Stem Cell Research (2007)

Trend 12. Do-It-Yourself Biotechnology

One of the most inspiring stories in science and biotechnology recently belongs to Jack Andraka. I met him in the Netherlands and in California, as we both gave speeches at the same events. Imagine a young teenager sitting in the cafeteria focusing on his upcoming speech but being kind to the many people who approach him only to say hello. He told me he had been interested in biosensing and learning about ways to detect environmental contaminants until the age of 13 when a close family friend who was like an uncle to him, passed away from pancreatic cancer.

He was confused, sad, and did not even know what a pancreas was, much less what pancreatic cancer was. He decided to turn to our era's simplest information resource, the Internet, to figure things out. His parents used to go to the library to do research and they told him of horror stories of spending hours looking in the card catalog and tracing down books only to find them missing from the collection.

He agrees with me that technology does connect us more now, and he was able to teach himself a lot because of the Internet, starting with Wikipedia, reading the bibliography and then the articles in those entries he was interested in. He printed out papers to read later in bed. He was taking a high school introduction to biology class in 8th grade when he had an epiphany moment:

"I was reading a paper on single walled carbon nanotubes while I was half listening to my teacher talk about antibodies. Suddenly I had an idea! What if I combined what I was reading about (nanotubes) with what I was supposed to be learning about (antibodies) and created a sensor to detect pancreatic cancer?"

Obviously, it was not that simple and he had lots more work to do, but thanks to modern technology he was able to learn what is needed to develop an experimental design. His mother told him a lab was definitely needed given that his design looked a lot more complicated than his previous experiments. He sent out many e-mails and got many rejections, which helped him learn to write better and more interesting messages. Finally, he got a chance to work under Anirban Maitra, Professor of Pathology at Johns Hopkins School of Medicine who was a huge inspiration to him.

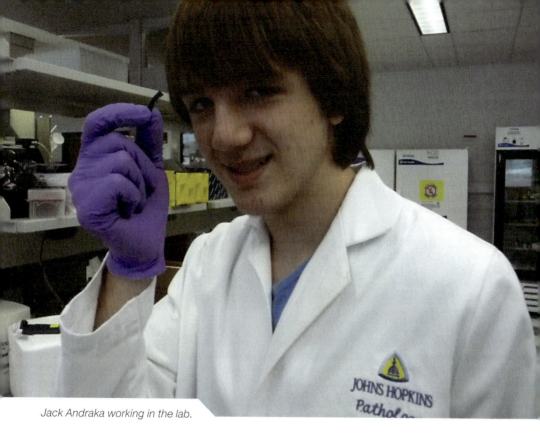

Jack Andraka working in the lab.

According to Andraka, the pancreatic cancer test he designed is 168 times faster, 1/26,000 as expensive (costing around three cents), and over 400 times more sensitive than the current diagnostic tests, and takes only five minutes to run. As a result, he won the 2012 Gordon E. Moore Award, the grand prize of the Intel International Science and Engineering Fair.

The method he worked out is truly innovative but has not been published yet in peer reviewed journals. Andraka discussed it with me saying that he was mostly concerned about seeing if the project would work; and after talking with his mentor and other high ranking scientists, he has learned that more work is needed before publication. Still, he cannot wait to move the project forward so the knowledge can help people. Currently, he is in talks with biotechnology companies to take over the work and further develop it.

He became an example for thousands of kids globally who have amazing ideas in science and medicine but do not want to go through the traditional (and slow) steps required. Instead, they try to find a solution right now by using all the connected opportunities they can find. Andraka answers questions from kids every day through e-mail and Skype and told me he loves

Trend 12. Do-It-Yourself Biotechnology

the energy, optimism, and excitement they bring to science and math. It is a great time to be a kid with big ideas because they are able to learn so much quickly and connect with one another and with experts easily. Mostly he tells them that if a 15 year old who did not even know what a pancreas was could create a sensor to detect cancer, just imagine what they can do.

He thinks it is important to keep raising awareness for more funding for research and to keep pushing for open access to scientific journals so that citizen scientists can learn and help innovate. After finishing high school, he hopes to attend a university and be able to continue researching and learning.

With fellow student Chloe Diggs, he recently took the $50,000 first prize in the Siemens "We Can Change the World Challenge" by developing a credit card–sized biosensor that can detect six environmental contaminants: mercury, lead, cadmium, copper, glyphosate, and atrazine. The idea came after learning about water pollution in a high school environmental science class. It costs $1 to make and takes 20 minutes to run, making it 200,000 times cheaper and 25 times more efficient than comparable sensors.

Jack Andraka meeting Barack Obama, President of the US.

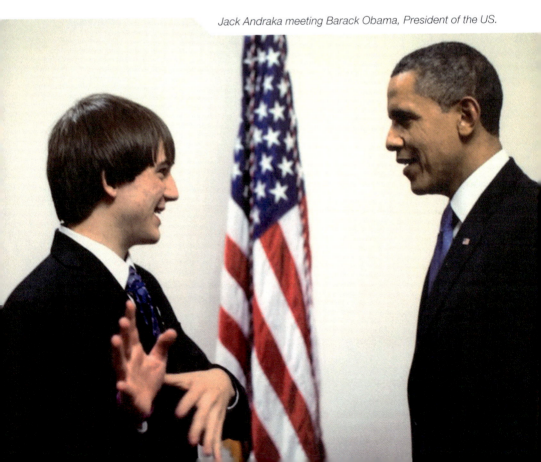

He is the perfect example how young scientists and science wannabes have the potential to contribute to research by simply having access to online databases, scientific information, and methods, as well as being open to innovation.

In a final example, and hopefully there will be more and more of these, Nathan Han won the Intel Science Fair in 2014 by developing an algorithm that is 81% accurate in identifying breast cancer-causing mutations, while the accuracy rate of existing algorithms is about 40%. The 15-year-old from Boston, US has been fascinated with bioinformatics, and chose to work out a new software for the mutation analysis of BRCA1, one of the most studied genes in the human genome, when a close friend's mother was diagnosed with ovarian cancer.

Biotechnology labs in the community

The first labs of the so-called Do-It-Yourself Biology community, a grassroots movement which was initiated to let students and others interested in biotechnology use professional laboratory equipment for their experiments, was launched in 2008. These enthusiasts seek to popularize biotechnology in the way that programmers popularized computing from their garages in the 1970s. Along with equipment, these labs provide a wellspring of biotech outreach and education. Local groups of DIY BIO are available from the US and Europe to Asia and Oceania.

BioCurious, a hackerspace for biotech, opened in 2011 with the mission statement that innovations in biology should be accessible, affordable, and open to everyone. They are building a community biology lab for amateurs, inventors, entrepreneurs, and anyone who wants to experiment with friends. They provide a complete working laboratory and technical library; equipment from fluorescent microscopes to PCR machines; materials; co-working space; and a training center for biotechniques. It was the first community biotech lab to crowdfund its start-up costs, the first to build a bioprinter, the first to sprout a company that Kickstarted almost half a million dollars. They are said to struggle with funding now, however.

The first time I came across The International Genetically Engineered Machine (iGEM) competition was when students working in the lab where I did my PhD decided to compete with one of their ideas. I learned that the Foundation behind iGEM is dedicated to education and competition, advancement of synthetic biology, and the development of open community and collaboration. It spun out of MIT in 2012 thus becoming an independent nonprofit organization

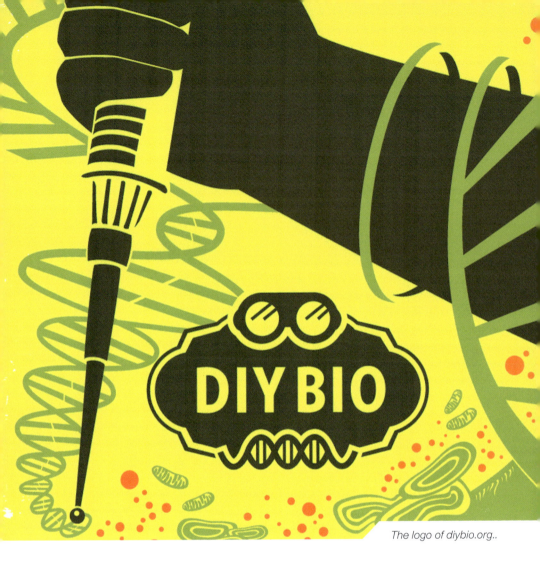

The logo of diybio.org..

located in Cambridge, Massachusetts. It began in January 2003 with a month-long course at MIT where students designed biological systems to make cells blink. It later grew to a summer competition with 5 teams in 2004, 13 teams in 2005, and gradually to 245 teams in 2012 and 2013.

Student teams are given a kit of biological parts at the beginning of the summer from the Registry of Standard Biological Parts. Working at their own schools, they use these parts and those of their own design to build biological systems and operate them in living cells. The project design and competition format provided an exceptionally motivating and effective teaching method. Students have created a rainbow of pigmented bacteria; an arsenic biodetector that responds to a range of arsenic concentrations in order to help under-developed countries detect arsenic contamination in water. They also developed BactoBlood, a cost-effective red blood cell substitute constructed from engineered bacteria. The system is designed to safely transport oxygen in the bloodstream without inducing sepsis, and to be stored for prolonged periods in a freeze-dried state. There is no limit to the teams' creativity.

Such community labs give youngsters interested in biotechnology and scientist wannabes a chance to test their ideas, conduct research, and get it to the final stage by making the results commercially available. This is the scenario that should be globally available to everyone with a good idea.

Biotech startups revolutionizing medicine

Elizabeth Holmes founded a company, Theranos, with her tuition money after dropping out of Stanford. The company develops a radical blood-testing service that requires only a pinprick and a drop of blood to perform hundreds of lab tests from standard cholesterol checks to sophisticated genetic analyses. This way, the results can be faster, more accurate, and cheaper than conventional methods. A motivation behind launching the company was her fear of needles, the only thing that actually scared her. Imagine how much more information such a test could provide if results would be better visualized and more informative. The same kind of data can be interpreted in different ways today due to the lack of quality in data visualizations.

Nanobiosym is dedicated to creating a new science that emerges from the holistic integration of physics, biomedicine, and nanotechnology. Examples include a portable nanotechnology platform that can rapidly and accurately detect genetic fingerprints from any biological organism, thus empowering people worldwide with rapid, affordable, and portable diagnostic information about their own health. The Cambridge, Massachusetts based company claims to have a diagnostic test that can detect the presence or absence of a disease's pathogen within an hour.

A company called uBiome is a microbiome sequencing service that provides information and tools for exploring microbiomes of customers who buy the service online. Based on research conducted the Human Microbiome Project, the company performs large-scale microbiome studies. Knowing the genomic background of our microbiome combined with our own genome and health information could yield a new way of identifying diseases and prescribing therapies.

Trend 12. Do-It-Yourself Biotechnology

Additionally, several recent studies focused on changing the basics of biology and taking biotechnology to the next level. Our DNA consists of 4 letters called nucleotides. In 2014, synthetic biologists at the Scripps Research Institute in La Jolla, California created cells with an expanded genetic alphabet that included two more letters, opening the door to a huge range of novel molecules. They have spent 15 years developing this new DNA whose sequences spell out instructions for making proteins. The next step is to determine whether cells can also transcribe the unnatural base pairs into RNA, and, ultimately, use them to make proteins.

At the same time, Autodesk, the design and engineering software company in California, created a synthetic bacteriophage, or virus, and then 3D printed the result. According to Andrew Hessel, an expert in this field, there is now the possibility that anyone can write software for living things with bio-code known as DNA. Completing the project took two weeks and about $1,000 compared to the multi-billion dollar efforts in the history of genomics.

Biotechnology has been one of the most promising areas of research in medicine, and it has not even shown its true potential. Re-thinking the basics of biology might have unknown consequences which we are not prepared for. The biotech industry has also been a key target for investors in the past couple of years, and it still could not take its deserved position, even though it has the potential to significantly change the way medicine is practiced through new solutions and by iterating the basics of biology.

Score of availability: 5
Focus of attention: Researchers
Websites & other online resources: iGEM (http://igem.org/), DIYBio (http://diybio.org/), BioCurious (http://biocurious.org/)
Companies & start-ups: Theranos (http://www.theranos.com/), Nanobiosym (http://www.nanobiosym.com/), uBiome (http://ubiome.com/)
Books: Culturing Life by Landecker, A Life Decoded by Venter; Life at the Speed of Light by Venter
Movies: Jurassic Park (1993)

Trend 13. The 3D Printing Revolution

A 14-month-old baby in the US had so many heart defects that it made the upcoming operation difficult. To better prepare in detail, hospital officials at Kosair Children's Hospital in Louisville, Kentucky contacted the J.B. Speed School of Engineering, where a polymer model of the baby's heart was created with a 3D printer. This provided vital insight ahead of surgery. Once the cardiothoracic surgeon had a model he knew exactly what he needed to do. The model allowed him to reduce the number of exploratory incisions and the overall operating time. This is just one example of how 3D printers could assist medical professionals.

3D printing fashions a three-dimensional object from a digital model by laying down successive layers of various materials. 3D printing could contribute to regenerative medicine, replacement surgery, operation planning, and many more ideas presented in this chapter.

Kaiba Gionfriddo was born prematurely in 2011. After 8 months his lung development caused concerns, although he was sent home with his parents as his breathing was normal. Six weeks later, Kaiba stopped breathing and turned blue. He was diagnosed with tracheobronchomalacia, a long Latin word that means his windpipe was so weak that it collapsed. He had a tracheostomy and was put on a ventilator––the conventional treatment. Still, Kaiba would stop breathing almost daily. His heart would stop, too. His caregivers 3D printed a bioresorbable device that instantly helped Kaiba breathe. This case is considered a prime example of how customized 3D printing is transforming healthcare as we know it.

In 2013 I spoke at Futuremed, which was organized by Singularity University. There I encountered 3D printing in person. I held a 3D-printed human jaw in my hands that had been printed out based on a patient's radiology scan.

Increasingly more objects can be made with 3D printers, and the biotechnology industry is keenly aware of the potential of this technology. Printing medical devices, living tissues, then eventually cells and pharmaceuticals might not be far away from everyday use. Parts such as bionic ears and simple organs might be printed at the patient's bedside, while printing transplantable human organs could eradicate waiting lists. Technological issues such as lack of available models or blueprints will be solved through crowdsourced and open-access databases from communities of designers.

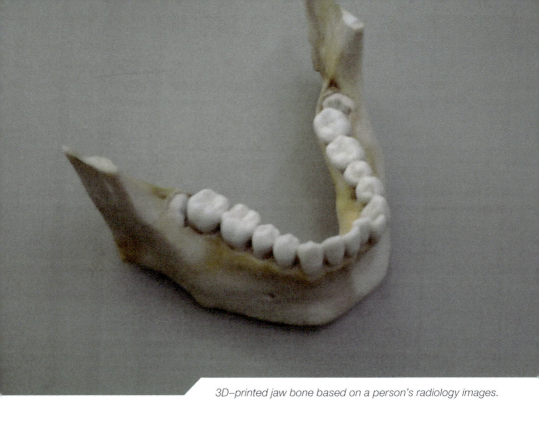

3D-printed jaw bone based on a person's radiology images.

3D printing to go mainstream

I've been following the articles of Michael Molitch-Hou for years. He's a Senior Writer at 3D Printing. He was one of the first experts I contacted to ask about this rapidly evolving industry.

"What I believe has really driven the 3D printing boom so far, though, is the open source movement around 3D printing that resulted from the expiration of important patents. Though Adrian Bowyer in the UK and Hod Lipson in the US were working on their open source 3D printers before the expiration of a key fused deposition modeling (FDM) patent owned by Scott Crump, inventor of FDM and founder of Stratasys, in 2009, it wasn't until after this patent expired that the movement exploded, fueling the entire 3D printing industry.

Once DIYers were making and, eventually commercializing their own 3D printers, they started to spread. They were way cheaper than any large manufacturer would have allowed and people could buy them in *kits and assemble their own for around $1,000 or so. Then, the media caught wind of it and, years later, you're writing a book that discusses how it impacts medicine."*

Therefore Molitch–Hou believes there needs to be a significant change in patent laws before the 3D printing industry can really take off. Imagine what would happen if pharmaceutical companies made the formulas for their drugs open source and publicly available, thereby allowing amateur scientists to synthesize medications, or small manufacturers to produce generic drugs at a fraction of the regular cost. If companies such as Organovo decided to release their designs as open source, than it might be possible for amateurs to 3D-print human tissues.

Aside from 3D-printed organs, he anticipates large, fast, multimaterial 3D printers to be invented soon. It could look like a single, robotic arm the size of a medium-sized construction vehicle. Or it could be an enormous gantry system able to extrude multiple materials. Molitch–Hou would also love to see electronic components entirely printed by 3D. If this were possible along with making 3D-printed metal components, we might be able to design a fully self-replicating 3D printer. The RepRap project was meant to explore possible designs for such a device. A preliminary study has already shown that using RepRaps to print common products results in economic savings.

The holy grail of 3D printing is printing molecules. If it were possible to determine the molecular makeup of an object and program it into the printer, we could produce endless copies of a living entity. Most likely we are not yet ready for that kind of development.

3D printing has grown from niche manufacturing to a $2.7 billion industry. As one of the key players of this new market, Organovo has over $24 million in equity precisely in order to attempt the manufacture of biomaterials and even artificial organs. Mike Renard in Commercial Operations spoke to me about their plans.

"We are working to provide better testing models for drug scientists with the goal to produce better and safer new medicines, at a lower total cost to develop. There are many stories of drugs failing too late in the discovery process, costing hundreds of millions of dollars with nothing to show for the effort. Moreover, there are examples of drugs that get to market, only to be recalled or restricted in their use because of life threatening complications for certain patients.

Trend 13. The 3D Printing Revolution

This area of science has great potential to be improved. Further, 18 people die each day in the US waiting for a possible life saving/extending tissue transplant. Other people live with a variety of chronic conditions due to various system failures, degenerative processes and metabolic deficiencies. The demand for functional tissue as a therapy alternative far exceeds the supply that will ever be available through current donor programs."

Printing living tissue compared to inanimate 3-dimensional objects is an enormous step even if technical improvements increasingly promise to make it a reality. Tissues in nature are three dimensional. They have defined architectures and repeating patterns. And they are made up of different cell types whose arrangement is critical to proper tissue function, as well as overall health of the system. 2D cell cultures and single cell lines are not capable of reproducing this complex native biology.

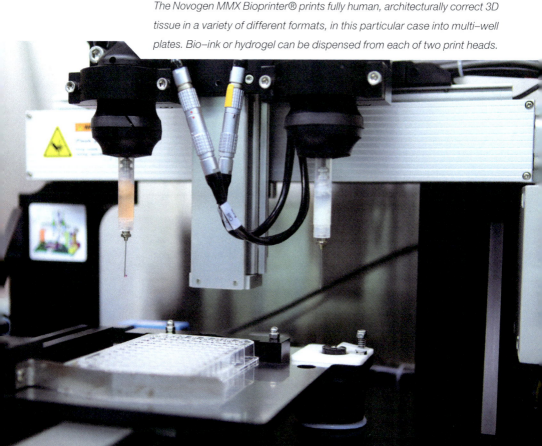

The Novogen MMX Bioprinter® prints fully human, architecturally correct 3D tissue in a variety of different formats, in this particular case into multi-well plates. Bio-ink or hydrogel can be dispensed from each of two print heads.

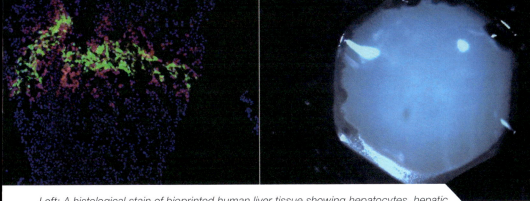

Left: A histological stain of bioprinted human liver tissue showing hepatocytes, hepatic stellate, and endothelial cells in an organized structure with the cell density and tight junctions of that found in native tissue. Right: Bioprinted human liver tissue in 3 dimensions.

Areas where printed living tissues could be used are expanding fast. One promising area is to create diseased tissues for research purposes. Having life-like disease models outside the body that behave like disease inside the body opens entirely new research avenues into the mechanisms of disease. These potential discoveries may fundamentally change how we target and design treatments, and how treatments may someday be personalized to an individual's phenotypic expression of a specific disease.

3D printing everything

The list of objects that have been successfully printed demonstrates the potential this technology holds for the near future.

Tissues with blood vessels: Researchers at Harvard University were the first to use a custom-built 3D printer and a dissolving ink to create a swatch of tissue that contains skin cells interwoven with structural material interwoven that can potentially function as blood vessels.

Low-Cost Prosthetic Parts: Creating traditional prosthetics is very time-consuming and destructive, which means that any modifications would destroy the original molds. Researchers at the University of Toronto, in collaboration with Autodesk Research and CBM Canada, used 3D printing to quickly produce cheap and easily customizable prosthetic sockets for patients in the developing world. Basically, they scan a damaged limb using Xbox Kinect, design the parts digitally, and then send the model to the printer which manufactures the socket in a few hours using polylactic acid, a thermoplastic

Trend 13. The 3D Printing Revolution

that is easily modifiable with heat. The cost with this method is under $10. If we merge 3D printing with open source templates that anyone can manufacture, distribute, and modify, then a new era of cheaper prosthetics for amputees around the world could begin.

Drugs: Lee Cronin, a chemist at the University of Glasgow, wants to do for the discovery and distribution of prescription drugs what Apple did for music. In a TED talk he described a prototype 3D printer capable of assembling chemical compounds at the molecular level. Patients would go to an online drugstore with their digital prescription, buy the blueprint and the chemical ink needed, and then print the drug at home. In the future he said we might sell not drugs but rather blueprints or apps. While this could make prescription drug distribution more efficient, a danger is that unscrupulous people will steal the designs and raw supplies in order to print out whatever drugs they want at home. This could become a regulatory nightmare, far worse than printing out guns. It will also restructure the pharmaceutical industry and biotechnology as we know it.

Tailor-made sensors: Researchers have used scans of animal hearts to create printed models, and then added stretchy electronics on top of those models. The material can be peeled off the printed model and wrapped around the real heart for a perfect fit. The next step is to enhance the electronics with multiple sensors. This demonstrates the promise of a new kind of personalized heart sensor.

Bone: Professor Susmita Bose of Washington State University modified a 3D printer to bind chemicals to a ceramic powder creating intricate ceramic scaffolds that promote the growth of the bone in any shape.

Heart Valve: Jonathan Butcher of Cornell University has printed a heart valve that will soon be tested in sheep. He used a combination of cells and biomaterials to control the valve's stiffness.

Ear cartilage: Lawrence Bonassar of Cornell University used 3D photos of human ears to create ear molds. The molds were then filled with a gel containing bovine cartilage cells suspended in collagen, which held the shape of the ear while cells grew their extracellular matrix.

Trend 13. The 3D Printing Revolution

Medical equipment: A clinic in Bolivia 140 kilometers from the nearest city prints out splints and prostheses when supplies are low. The cost per piece runs about 2 cents for the plastic. This might allow developing nations to circumvent having to import large numbers of supplies. Already, 3D printing is occurring in underdeveloped areas. "Not Impossible Labs" based in Venice, California took 3D printers to Sudan where the chaos of war has left many people with amputated limbs. The organization's founder, Mick Ebeling, trained locals how to operate the machinery, create patient-specific limbs, and fit these new, very inexpensive prosthetics.

Tamperproof cable tether: Biomedical technician Steven Jaworski at Brookhaven Memorial Hospital designed a cable tether that holds together huge amount of wires and printed it out 3D using Makerbot, saving the hospital considerable money.

Cranium Replacement: Dutch surgeons replaced the entire top of a 22 year-old woman's skull with a customized printed implant made from plastic.

Tumor Models: Researchers in China and the US have both printed models of cancerous tumors to aid discovery of new anti-cancer drugs and to better understand how tumors develop, grow, and spread.

Eye: Fripp Design and Research in the United Kingdom aims to print out 150 prosthetic eyes in an hour. Mass production not only promised to speed up the manufacture of eye prostheses, but also significantly lower the costs. Additionally, customers can choose the color of the prosthesis.

Synthetic skin: James Yoo at the Wake Forest School of Medicine in the US has developed a printer that can print skin straight onto the wounds of burn victims.

Organs: Organovo announced in 2013 that their bioprinted liver assays were able to function for more than 40 days. Organovo's top executives and other industry experts suggest that within a decade we will be able to print solid organs such as liver, heart, and kidney. Hundreds of thousands of people worldwide are waiting for an organ donor. Imagine how such a technology could transform their lives.

Trend 13. The 3D Printing Revolution

To illustrate the big picture Molitch–Hou shared with me the story of Liam, a US child born with amniotic band syndrome. This results in only the partial formation of the fingers. Meanwhile, in South Africa, a woodworker named Richard Van As had his fingers severed in a woodworking accident. Both faced the costs of modern prosthetics, which for Richard might be $10,000 for a finger alone.

Elsewhere, an automation technician named Ivan Owen posted a YouTube video of a mechanical hand prop he had made for Halloween. Richard came across the video and subsequently asked if Ivan could construct a prosthetic arm with fingers for him. Living on opposite sides of the globe they communicated by Skype. MakerBot donated a MakerBot Replicator to each of them, which allowed them to print iterations of their prosthetic prototypes back and forth to each other until Richard got a good fit.

When Liam's father heard about their project he asked Ivan and Richard to help him construct a prosthetic hand for his son. After trial and error, Liam's dad was able to 3D print a set of plastic fingers good enough to grasp

A boy with a cheap prosthetic device printed out in 3D with RoboHand.

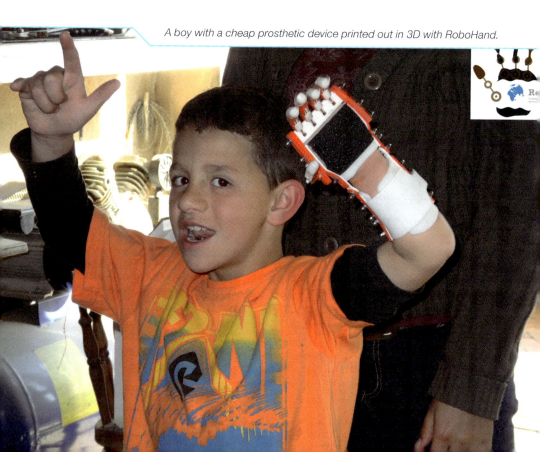

Trend 13. The 3D Printing Revolution

objects. This story of prosthetic hands has since become widespread, so much that Richard has started an organization called RoboHand that works to help people like Liam and himself print affordable prosthetics. RoboHand has begun developing a low-cost printed leg prosthesis. Richard has even worked with "Not Impossible Labs" and his efforts have inspired other organizations, such as e-Nable, to also pursue the 3D prosthesis printing.

The key here is the price difference of prosthetics created by different methods. For the cost of a myoelectric device that take signals from muscle fibers in the arm and send them to the fingers, one can print out 840 3D hands. Robohand has already enabled 200 people to use these inexpensive but very functional prosthetics. Its designs are obviously open source. 3D printing will soon be mainstream. The concept shows how it can revolutionize several elements of worldwide healthcare so long as regulatory and technical difficulties can be overcome.

Score of availability: 4

Focus of attention: Patients and medical professionals

Websites & other online resources: 3D Printing News (http://3dprintingindustry.com/medical/), The Cronin Group (http://www.chem.gla.ac.uk/cronin/)

Companies & start-ups: MakerBot (http://www.makerbot.com/), 3Dsystems (http://www.3dsystems.com/)

Books: MAKE, Ultimate Guide to 3D Printing 2014 by Frauenfelder

Movies: Iron Man 2 (2010)

Trend 14. Iron Man: Powered exoskeletons and prosthetics

On a sunny day in November, 2013 I attended the Europe Summit organized by the Singularity University in Budapest at the amazing venue of the Franz Liszt Academy of Music. We listened to Amanda Boxtel, who got paralyzed from a spinal cord injury in a ski accident in Aspen, Colorado in 1992. She told us how she felt after getting the diagnosis of never being able to walk again and how she refused to stop dreaming. Since then, she has established adaptive ski programs, carried the Olympic torch, organized disabled rafting expeditions, and even conducted research in the Antarctica. She has also become one of the ambassadors of an innovative company called Ekso Bionics.

Ekso Bionics was launched in California in 2005 with a brave mission to design and develop powered exoskeletons that could make walking possible again for paralyzed people. A powered exoskeleton is a mobile framework that a person wears. It contains motors or hydraulics that deliver part of the energy needed for limb movement.

Their exoskeletons are used by individuals with various degrees of paralysis and stemming by a variety of causes. By the end of 2012 Ekso Bionics had helped individuals take more than a million steps that would not otherwise have been possible. Boxtel is one of ten Ekso Bionics test pilots who received a customized exoskeleton. According to Boxtel, the project "represents the triumph of human creativity and technology that converged to restore my authentic functionality in a stunningly beautiful, fashionable and organic design."

The exoskeleton she wore at the conference was custom designed using precision 3D printing. Body scans helped the designers mold the robotic suit to her measurement. They then coupled the suit with mechanical parts and controls. This process usually takes about three months.

Designers had to face various challenges, such as whether paralyzed people can feel or not because undetected bruises can become infected. Boxtel's suit which was designed to fit her body with Velcro straps. This allows her skin to breathe so that she can walk without sweating too much.

Other challenges included the problem of power supply, joint flexibility, error control to detect invalid movements, and customization. Yet what better to illustrate the progress made than to have an individual in an exoskeleton making the kick–off at the football World Cup taking place in Brazil in 2014?

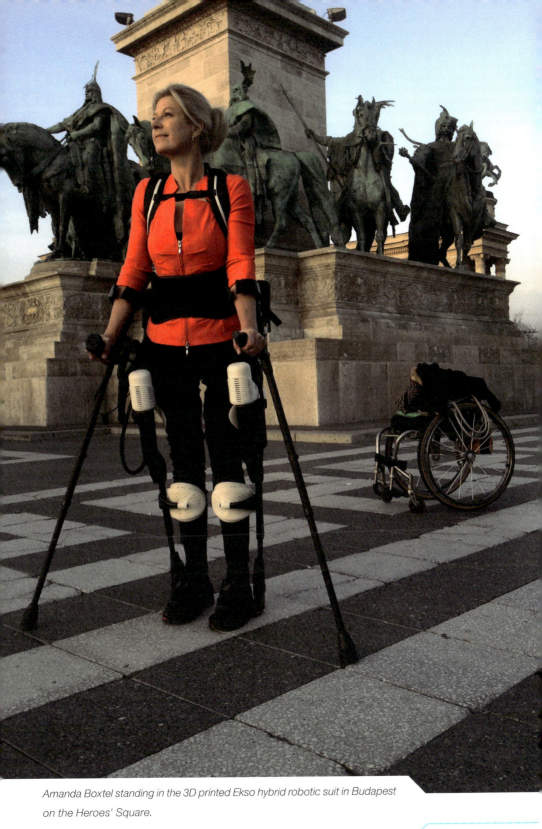

Amanda Boxtel standing in the 3D printed Ekso hybrid robotic suit in Budapest on the Heroes' Square.

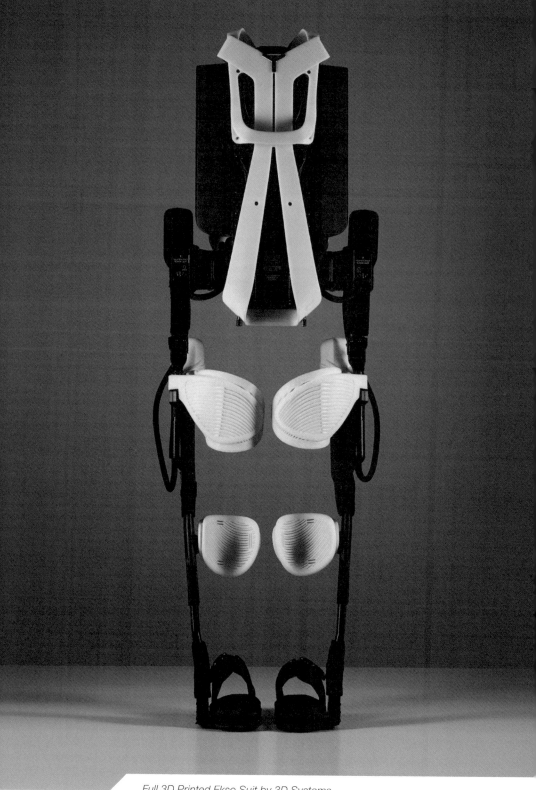
Full 3D Printed Ekso Suit by 3D Systems.

Trend 14. Iron Man: Powered exoskeletons and prosthetics

I discussed the future of Ekso Bionics with its Chief Technology Officer, Russ Angold. He has held assorted engineering positions at several companies, and works closely with the Lockheed Martin Corporation in licensing Ekso technology. He described the huge attention around the product:

"It is really interesting that we had over 3000 different individuals in our database in less than 2 years. The device is helping a lot of people who otherwise could not work, or their therapy would take a long time. Our job is giving them the technology that allows them to stay healthy and live a full life."

Ekso Bionics is working to make its technology available to more individuals ever since it started focusing on spinal cord injury. They now want to expand it to other conditions; and even add developments therefore the device could accommodate to those patients who have, for instance, 100% strength on one side and paralysis on the other. In considering cost one must factor in its value in reducing secondary complications such as urinary infections or chronic pain.

Angold pointed out that any new technology faces obstacles, and that paralysis can be emotionally trying for patients. While the company is careful not to overpromise what the device can do, they are working to gain great acceptance among medical professionals and patients who can benefit from their exoskeletons.

Architect Robert Woo had an accident that left him quadriplegic. His arms recovered in time, but both legs remained paralyzed. He felt useless and wanted to die. Turning to the Internet he came across a robotic exoskeleton called ReWalk developed by Argo Medical Technologies in Israel. He applied for their research program and trained in their use. Typical patients need twenty to seventy sessions to learn how to use these wearable robots. Woo mentioned how thrilling it was to be able to again stand next to his wife and give her a hug, and to walk with his children to the park. These are things that people take for granted, but which he has missed very much.

Italian engineers at the Perceptual Robotics Laboratory developed what they called a Body Extender, a robot that can help move heavy objects as an exoskeleton by lifting about 50 kilograms in each of its hands. It is claimed to be the most complex exoskeleton yet built. It can be used for assembling complicated products such as aircrafts; rescue victims after an earthquake or moving rocks away. We have not even begun to see the real potential of exoskeletons.

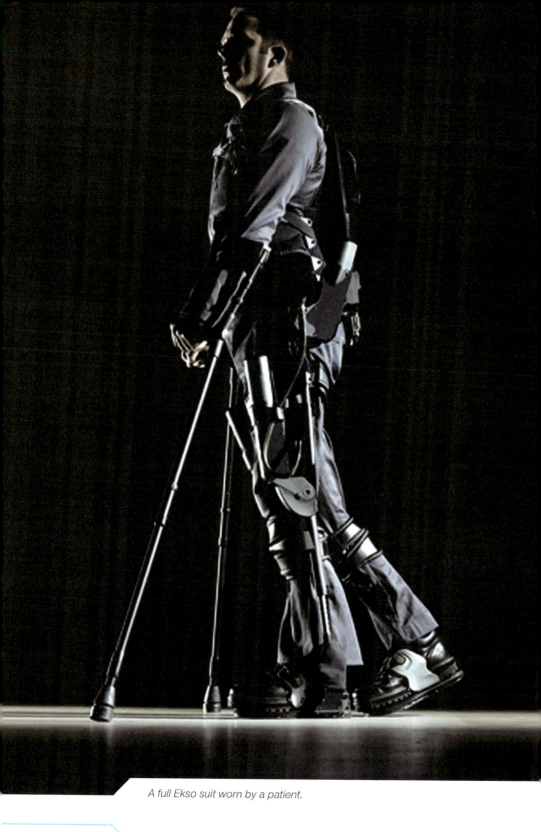
A full Ekso suit worn by a patient.

Customizing prosthetics

Hugh Herr, who directs the Biomechatronics research group at MIT's Media Lab, gave an amazing TED talk in 2014. Herr lost both his legs in a climbing accident 30 years earlier. He spoke of his plan to make flexible, smart prosthetics cheaper and widely available for those who need them. His team is pioneering a new class of smart biohybrid prostheses and exoskeletons for people with physical disabilities. It builds prosthetic knees, legs, and ankles that fuse biomechanics with microprocessors in order to restore normal gait, balance, and speed. They may even enhance biological functions including strength or speed. At the end of his talk came a surprise. Ballroom dancer Adrianne Haslet–Davis, who lost her left leg in the 2013 Boston Marathon bombing, performed on stage for us for the first time since her accident.

The Rehabilitation Institute of Chicago (RIC), designers at Vanderbilt University and prosthetics company Freedom Innovations reached a breakthrough by creating artificial limbs that allow amputees to walk up stairs, rotate an ankle, and navigate sloped terrains merely by thinking about it. A brain–controlled bionic leg is clearly a huge step in the future. RIC has been working on this since 2005. Using their innovation in 2012, Zac Vawter climbed over 2000 steps to the 103rd floor of Chicago's Willis Tower after losing his leg four years earlier in a motorcycle accident.

In 2014, the prosthetic won FDA approval for use in rehabilitation facilities, but not yet for personal use at home. Companies, researchers, and patients are petitioning the FDA to approve home use as well.

A San Francisco based company, Bespoke Innovations, went further in customization to make beautifully designed prosthetics based on the patient's needs and personality. Scott Summit, the designer at Bespoke, explained that in single amputees, the remaining leg is scanned and mirrored to give the correct geometry.

Athlete Jozef Metelka lost his leg in a 2009 motorbike accident and now has 12 different prosthetics that serve different functions from mountain biking and skiing to snowboarding and rollerblading. Each was designed by specialists at Pace Rehabilitation in the United Kingdom.

Another athlete, Mike Schultz, was a top professional snowmobile racer when his accident resulted in an amputation above the knee. With the help of the FOX Company that makes shock absorbers and racing suspensions, he designed and manufactured the prototype of the so–called "Moto Knee".

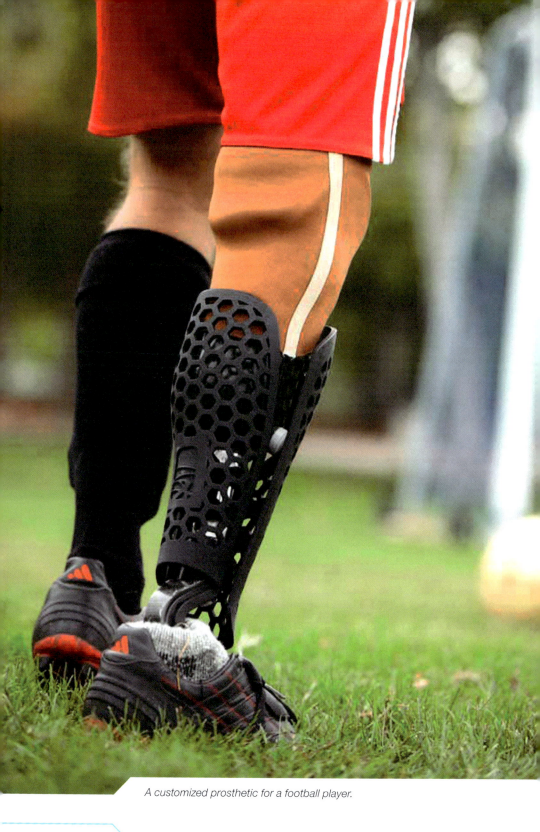
A customized prosthetic for a football player.

Trend 14. Iron Man: Powered exoskeletons and prosthetics

He later won multiple X–Games Gold Medals in the adaptive snow cross and motocross categories by using his own invention. The company he founded, Biodapt, sold over 100 of his extreme–sports prosthetics to other amputees so they could get back into the games they loved.

The real challenge for such companies is to design devices that can almost perfectly mimic the complex movements of hands and legs. Based on their i–limb technology, Touch Bionics introduced a prosthetic hand that allows individual fingers to move independently. Not only can the thumb rotate, but an iPhone app lets users control grip patterns as well. By clicking on the screen they can choose whatever grip patterns they prefer to use a mouse or to type, for instance. Life becomes much easier.

A photo from 1890 shows a little girl with prosthetic legs that seemed to be too modern compared to the technological advancements of that time. Many thought the photo was a hoax, but the photo was credited to James Gillingham, a well–respected shoemaker in 19th century England. He began making artificial limbs after a local man lost his arm in 1863. It is stunning how much this area has developed since then. And the end is not even near.

A customized prosthetic for a man who likes to ride his motorcycle.

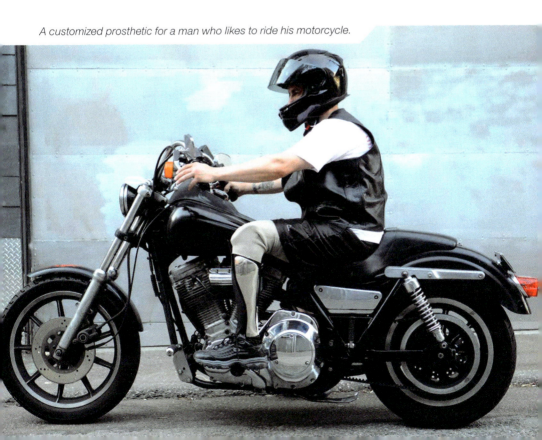

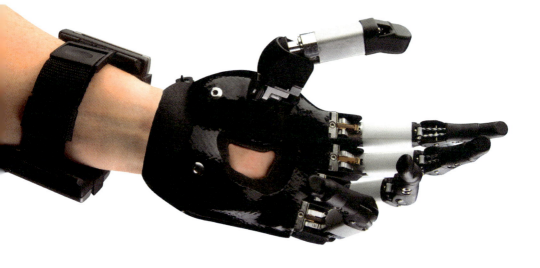

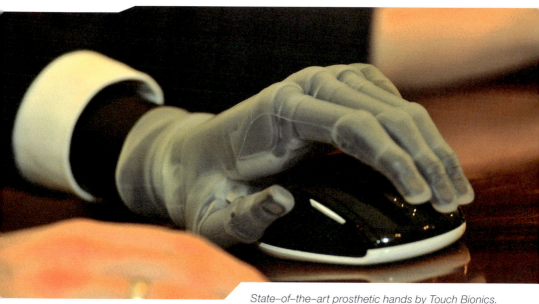

State-of-the-art prosthetic hands by Touch Bionics.

Neuroprosthetics

The ultimate goal is to make touch-sensitive prosthetic limbs that provide its wearer with real-time information via a direct interface with the brain. In one study, researchers identified brain patterns of neural activity that occur during natural object manipulation, and managed to induce the same areas by artificial manipulation. An interdisciplinary team of experts from academic institutions, government agencies, and private companies work on creating prosthetics that would restore natural motor control and sensation as a part of Revolutionizing Prosthetics, a DARPA project.

Trend 14. Iron Man: Powered exoskeletons and prosthetics

Something similar happened in the movie "The Empire Strikes Back" as Luke Skywalker received a complete prosthetic arm with a sense of touch after losing his arm in a battle.

Dennis Aabo Sørensen who lost his left hand in a fireworks explosion many years ago could tell what he was touching with his prosthetic hand again at the age of 36 because now it is possible to attach wired pressure sensors in the fingers of an artificial hand to sensory nerves in the upper arm. He could feel the shape and surface texture of the objects he touched. His first reaction was amazement at being able to feel something he had not felt in many years.

Medical professionals and engineers at the RIC have developed artificial limbs that can respond to a patient's thoughts. Computer chips implanted into the prosthetic limb are connected to sensors that pick up motor signals from the nerves that formerly made the hand move. To accomplish this, surgeons first had to reroute the nerves to large muscles at the end of the stump so that those muscles amplify the nerve signals. The strengthened nerve signals can then be detected by the prosthetic sensors which send them to motors that move the hand.

The ethical dilemmas

Bertolt Meyer, an academic known as "the bionic man," has had a cutting-edge £40,000 artificial forearm and hand since 2009. In 2013, he raised concerns about scientists and engineers launching technological advances on the open market without a prior ethical debate. He fears that who can afford it will be unfairly augmented and have an advantage over those who cannot. When this becomes apparent to everyone, he thinks a mass market for bionic enhancement will develop.

Meyer authored the documentary "How to Build a Bionic Man", in which he reveals how his own old prosthesis made him feel ashamed, while the newer one gives him confidence when out in public.

What happens to society when such artificial limbs start to offer truly augmented human capabilities? An example for this is the case of Professor Gil Weinberg who has created a robotic drumming prosthesis that can be attached to amputees. A drummer who now wears this additional drumstick can use the prosthesis and make it improvise while he is playing.

Trend 14. Iron Man: Powered exoskeletons and prosthetics

Another example is Matthew James, born with dysmelia, a congenital disorder causing deformed limbs. James wrote to his favorite Formula One team, Mercedes, at age 14 that he was ready to display their logo on his prosthesis if they could support him financially. He received £30,000 but was not taken up on his offer of advertising space. This story shows that the implementation of such innovations in the everyday lives cannot depend purely on individual entrepreneurship.

These devices are extremely expensive at the moment. Jose Delgado Jr. was born without a left hand. His health insurance covered the cost of a $42,000 myoelectric device. He recently received an offer from 3DUniverse to print out a Cyborg Beast prosthetic hand. Such open source printed hands are used in the Robohand project as well. Delgado was surprised that the 3D hand turned out to function better than the myoelectric device, so he decided to keep using it. It is true that the plastic used in 3D printing is easy to break, but it is a simple matter to print out a new one. The cost is almost nothing compared to conventional prosthetics.

Being born without a limb or losing one in an accident will soon not be a major disadvantage. As technology improves at a fast rate, these may even augment normal human capabilities. The real question facing us is not whether technology will be able to help such patients, but how to persuade healthy people in the near future not to change their own limbs to smart, state-of-the-art prosthetics.

Score of availability: 4
Focus of attention: Patients
Websites & other online resources: International Society for Prosthetics and Orthotics (http://www.ispoint.org/)
Companies & start-ups: Bespoke Innovations (http://www.bespokeinnovations.com/), Robohand (http://www.robohand.net/), Ekso Bionics (http://eksobionics.com)
Books: Powered exoskeleton 39 Success Secrets: 39 Most Asked Questions On Powered exoskeleton – What You Need To Know Paperback –by Horn
Movies: The Matrix Reloaded (2003), Avatar (2009), Iron Man 2 (2010), Elysium (2013), Edge of Tomorrow (2014)

Trend 15. The End of Human Experimentation

Today, new pharmaceuticals are approved by a process that culminates in human clinical trials. The clinical trial is a rigorous process from development of the active molecule to animal trials before the human ones, costing billions of dollars and requiring many years. Patients participating in the trial are exposed to side effects, not all of which will have been predicted by animal testing. If the drug is successful in trial, it may receive approval, but the time and expense are present regardless of the trial outcome.

But what if there were another, safer, faster, and less expensive route to approval? Instead of requiring years of "ex vivo" and animal studies before human testing, what if it were possible to test thousands of new molecules on billions of virtual patients in just a few minutes? What would be required to demonstrate such a capability? At the very least, the virtual patients must mimic the physiology of the target patients, with all of the variation that actual patients show. The model should encompass circulatory, neural, endocrine, and metabolic systems, and each of these must demonstrate valid mechanism–based responses to physiological and pharmacological stimuli. The model must also be cost efficient, simulating weeks in a span of seconds.

Such simulations are called computational cognitive architectures, although the current ones actually lack a comprehensive representation of human physiology. A truly comprehensive system would make it possible to model conditions, symptoms, and even drug effects. To order reach this brave goal, every tiny detail of the human body needs to be included in the simulation from the way our body reacts to temperature changes to the circadian rhythms of hormone action.

HumMod is a simulation system that provides a top–down model of human physiology from organs to hormones. It now contains over 1,500 linear and non–linear equations and over 6,500 state variables such as body fluids, circulation, electrolytes, hormones, metabolism, and skin temperature. HumMod was based on original work by Drs. Arthur Guyton and Thomas Coleman in the early 1970's.

Over the last forty years Coleman has taken their work and expanded it, first with a DOS based program called Human, then as a Windows based one called Quantitative Circulatory Physiology which is freely available and written in C++ programming language which made coding physiology challenging. Over the last eight years Dr. Robert Hester has directed the

Trend 15. The End of Human Experimentation

development of HumMod in tackling such issues, and now the physiology component is written in a format called XML.

Researchers' focus has been to create HumMod People, a population model of HumMod that allows for the simulation of "humans" with different physiological responses. This work can potentially help us understand how a human population responds differently to certain pathologies or drugs. Ongoing research in this field suggests that it will soon be possible to mimic the human body in simulation. I contacted Hester to get his expert opinion.

"We believe that there is a major problem with the way that physiological models have been developed. Our methods have been to start at a top level, with what may be considered initial crude descriptions of the physiological pathways. Then we add detail to these "crude" mathematical descriptions, thus refining the model. The benefit of this is that we develop an integrative model of human physiology. Other designs start at a lower level, such as biochemical and molecular simulation, and try to fit these models together. We believe there are several challenges with this type of simulation. One is that there is not sufficient experimental human data that will allow one to understand the biochemical pathways under a variety of conditions."

In the last few months they have been working with a company developing a device to monitor congestive heart failure in an attempt to predict when the patient should see their physician rather than go to an Emergency Room or be admitted to the hospital. Their patient model has a variety of pathologies and has generated simulations over a two–month period of operation. The company compared the resulting data to the human data to determine whether they were collecting the appropriate parameters.

HumMod was licensed from the University of Mississippi to commercialize the software and get funding to continue the project. It is now turning in different directions. The first is medical education. A browser version of HumMod is being developed to help students at all levels understand basic physiology. Programming patient scenarios and implementing HumMod into medical mannequins to provide realistic physiological responses can better train medical and nursing students to manage patients for the long term. Conducting physiological and clinical research is another obvious application.

As Dr. Hester indicated, the implementation of personalized medicine would certainly require such a physiological model.

Trend 15. The End of Human Experimentation

"The idea that each of us is just like the other and should be treated (clinically) like anyone else is obsolete now. If our assumption is correct, that the equations underlying physiology are sacrosanct but that the coefficients (parameters) capture the differences in individuals. With a large enough "library" of patients, observations from a single patient can marginalize the library to a similar population. As observation continues, the larger pool might be winnowed down to a "most expressive" model, which might then be used as a basis for planning treatment, diet, exercise regimen, or any other aspect of health. The idea, while years from any kind of implementation, is intuitively clear."

Many elements from energy balance to neural signals still need improvement in order to make HumMod capable of simulating chronic conditions and complicated protocols. Generating large data sets will require appropriate software for proper analyses, but beyond these issues the long-term goal of the HumMod project is to model human physiology from birth to death.

HumMod is not the only effort in this area. The Avicenna project, partially funded by the European Commission, aims to construct a roadmap for future "in silico" clinical trials, which would make it possible to conduct them without actually experimenting on people. Other projects use real models instead of computational ones. A liver human organ construct, a physical object that responds to toxic chemical exposure the way a real liver does, was designed at the Gordon A. Cain University. The goal of the five-year, $19 million multiinstitutional project is to develop interconnected human organ constructs that are based on a miniaturized platform nicknamed ATHENA (Advanced Tissue-engineered Human Ectypal Network Analyzer) that looks like a CPR mannequin.

It would then be possible to test molecules without risking the toxic effects on humans, and to monitor fluctuations in the thousands of different molecules that living cells produce and consume. The beauty of this project is its plan to connect their working liver device to a heart device developed by Harvard University. If successful, they hope to add a lung construct in 2015 that is being developed at Los Alamos, and a kidney designed by the UCSF/Vanderbilt collaboration by 2016, thus building the first physiological model of a human being piece by piece.

Trend 15. The End of Human Experimentation

Simulating organs on chips

Simulating human physiology does not necessarily require building organs the same size as living human ones. Their physiology can be modeled more easily. A technique called organ–on–a–chip simulates the activities, mechanics, and physiology of entire organs and organ systems. An individual organ–on–chip is composed of a clear flexible polymer the size of a computer memory stick that contains hollow microfluidic channels lined by living human cells. The chips provide a literal glimpse into the inner workings of human organs given the transparent nature of the microdevices. Organs and structures including heart, lung, kidney, artery, bone, cartilage, and skin have been simulated by microfluidic

Designing a whole body biomimetic device will potentially correct one of the most significant limitations on organs–on–chips: the isolation of organs.

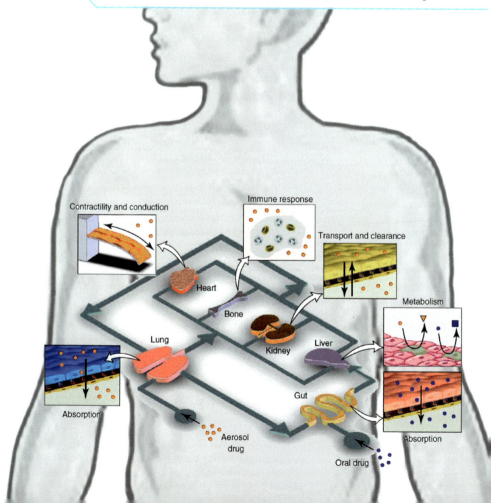

devices. They can let pharmaceutical companies measure direct effects of one organ's reaction on another. However, because the system becomes more complex as the design expands, as do the challenges that grow with it.

The Wyss Institute and a team of collaborators seek to link ten human organs–on–chips to imitate whole–body physiology. The instrument will control fluid flow and cell viability while permitting real–time observation of the cultured tissues and analysis of complex biochemical functions. This instrument will be called human–on–a–chip. It could be used to assess new drug candidates and provide critical information on their safety and efficacy. In 2014, the Wyss Institute created a bone–marrow–on–a–chip that reproduces the structure, function, and even cellular make–up of this complex human tissue. It will be a test tool for researchers studying the effects and toxicity of new drugs. Moreover, it could be used to maintain a cancer patient's bone marrow temporarily while undergoing radiation or chemotherapy that commonly destroys the tissue.

A revolutionary aspect of this new bone–marrow–on–a–chip is that it can actually generate blood cells in an artificial circulatory system which itself could supply the network of other organs–on–chips. Both the FDA and DARPA have provided funding for these efforts. Ultimately such devices could replace animal testing of new drugs and environmental toxins as well as accurately modeling human diseases.

Organ–specific features that can be modulated in human physiological models.

Organ	Demonstrated organ-specific features
Liver	Serum protein synthesis, liver zonation
Lung	Airway closure and opening, inflammation, alveolar-capillary interface
Kidney	Molecular transport
Gut	Intestinal absorption
Bone	Lacuna-canicular network
Breast	Cancer metastasis
Brain	Formation of new blood vessels in tumors

Trend 15. The End of Human Experimentation

Another example from Georgia Institute of Technology is a device that mimics blood flow through narrowed coronary arteries in order to assess the effects of anti–clotting drugs such as aspirin. A study concluded that while aspirin can prevent dangerous blood clots in some patients at risk for thrombosis, it may not be effective in those merely with narrowed arteries. Given that doctors have a huge range of drugs from which to choose, such benchtop diagnostic devices could help save lives by preventing heart attacks while also lowering healthcare costs.

In 2014 tissue containing an individual's specific genetic disorder was replicated in the laboratory for the first time. Harvard scientists in collaboration with the Wyss Institute and others obtained skin cells from a patient with Barth syndrome, a rare cardiac disorder for which there is no known cure. They transformed the skin cells into stem cells that carried the mutation by using chips with human extracellular matrix proteins that mimicked the natural environment. The heart tissue grew out of these cells produced only weak contractions similarly to the weak heart muscle in Barth's syndrome. They concluded that we cannot really understand the meaning of a single cell's genetic mutation until a large chunk of organ is built and makes it possible to see how it functions or malfunctions.

Microengineered cell–culture systems mimicking organ physiology can be used to develop disease models that are relevant to people and more predictive of drug efficacy and toxicity while also providing better insights into the mechanism of drug action. We might discover new routes of drug delivery; analyze populations with different genetic backgrounds; determine pharmacokinetic properties of various compounds; even conduct clinical trials using microengineered models.

In 2014, the Insigneo Institute built a fully computer–simulated model of human physiology for personalized healthcare. "The Virtual Physiological Human" is intended to circumvent issues of clinical trials and animal testing by simulating the outcomes of therapies for patients. What they are working on could be vital to the future of healthcare. Without in silico medicine, organizations will be unable to cope with future demand. The Virtual Physiological Human will be a software–based laboratory for experimentation and treatment that can save time and money and lead to superior treatment outcomes.

Trend 15. The End of Human Experimentation

If all the data on a patient were added to their simulation, it could make predictions about the given individual's status and future health outcomes, thus ushering in an era of truly individualized medicine. The team is also working on VIRTUheart for assessing coronary artery disease, a neuromuscular model for predicting treatment for Parkinson's disease, MySpine focusing on disc degeneration, and Mission–T2D that models a patient's risk of developing type 2 diabetes.

These examples show that an in–silico human is not going to appear in the next few years, but only in the distant future. We might not have the chance in our lifetimes of having simulated copies of ourselves model the illnesses we will develop. If we had them now, we could stop human experiments with new drugs and compounds that might be toxic; stop using animals during early stages of such trials; be able to predict treatment outcomes and the onset of disease before symptoms develop. All this would lead to a revolution in healthcare from the perspective of decreased costs and saving lives with computer models.

Score of availability: 2
Focus of attention: Researchers
Websites & other online resources: The Wyss Institute (http://wyss.harvard.edu/), Hummod (http://hummod.org/), Avicenna (http://avicenna–isct.org/)
Companies & start–ups: Virtual Physiology (http://www.virtual–physiology.com/)
Books: Handbook of Virtual Humans by Thalmann & Thalmann
Movies: S1m0ne (2002), The Congress (2013)

Trend 16. Medical Decisions via Artificial Intelligence

In 2011, people witnessed an interesting and at the same time weird competition on the television quiz show Jeopardy. It featured the two best players in the history of the show, Ken Jennings, who had the longest unbeaten run of 74 winning appearances, and Brad Rutter, who had earned the biggest prize of $3.25 million. Their opponent was a huge computer with over 750 servers and a cooling system stored at a location so as not to disturb the players. The room–sized machine was made by IBM and named after the company's founder, Thomas J. Watson. It did not smile or show emotion, but it kept on giving good answers. At the end, Watson won the game with $77,147 leaving Rutter and Jennings with $21,600 and $24,000 respectively.

Watson is perhaps the most important supercomputer, and one of the first to enter the artificial intelligence (AI) market in our time. Its success depends on how it acquires new knowledge. Martin Kohn, medical director of IBM Watson, explains that its training is an ongoing process, and it is rapidly improving its ability to render reasonable recommendations that oncologists, for example, think are helpful. Watson is also said to ascertain quickly what it does not yet know. Siri, the intelligent assistant in Apple's iOS, on the other hand, simply looks for keywords to search the web, and lists options from which one can choose.

What even the most acclaimed professors know cannot match cognitive computers. As the amount of information they accumulate grows exponentially, the assistance of computing solutions in medical decisions is imminent. While a physician can keep a few dozen study results and papers in mind, IBM's Watson can process more than 200 million pages in seconds. This remarkable speed has led to trying Watson in oncology centers to see how helpful it is in making treatment decisions in cancer care. Watson does not answer medical questions, but based on data it comes up with the most relevant and likely outcomes. Physicians make the final call. Computer assistance can only facilitate the work of physicians, not replace it.

IBM's chief of research said that what first hit them about Watson was its list of endless opportunities, because as the concept it represents can be applied to almost any situation. Initially the team chose medicine for obvious reasons. Imagine how useful Watson could be by suggesting diagnoses and treatment options. Watson could be the perfect tool to navigate decision trees

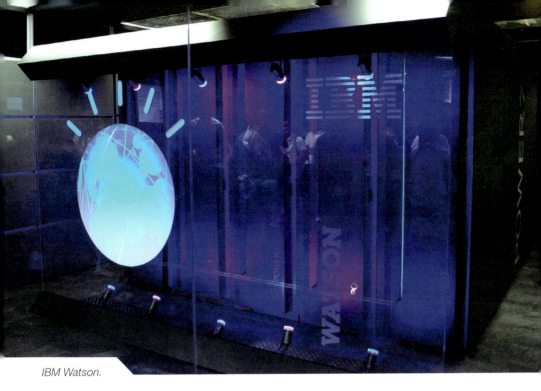

IBM Watson.

used by cancer specialists that weigh treatment options involving radiation, surgery, and countless numbers of chemotherapy drugs. It can read the world's medical journals, digest patient histories, keep an eye on the latest drug trials and new therapies, and even state-of-the-art guidelines in less time than it takes a physician to drink a cup of coffee. And it constantly keeps on learning.

    Not surprisingly Watson has been tested in 2012 in different settings such as the Memorial Sloan Kettering Cancer Center. Simultaneously, Wellpoint, a large health insurer in the US, began using a Watson computer to speed up the authorization of medical procedures. Sometimes they refer to this transition as Watsonizing.

    Watson's work with clinicians demonstrates how it could potentially transform healthcare. For more than a year, Watson has been trained in science and medicine by feeding it medical textbooks, peer reviewed journals, patient histories, and treatment guidelines. At Memorial Sloan-Kettering doctors used a tablet application to access the computer through the cloud. They input data or ask questions. Because Watson understands natural language, a query about a cancer treatment, for example, makes Watson note keywords, the particular type of cancer, and the genomic variant of the tumor. Using massively parallel processors, Watson then reviews millions of relevant pages

Trend 16. Medical Decisions via Artificial Intelligence

of text, studies, patient's history, and much more in seconds. It generates hypotheses for treatment, suggesting options with varying levels of confidence on the tablet app. The doctor then makes the call by weighing the options.

According to Sloan–Kettering, it would take at least 160 hours of weekly reading just to keep up with the medical literature. As a result only around 20% of what doctors use when diagnosing and deciding on treatments relies on trial–based evidence. As Wellpoint officials noted, Watson's correct diagnosis rate for lung cancer is 90%, compared to 50% for human doctors.

Herbert Chase, a professor of clinical medicine at Columbia University who consulted with IBM during the development of Watson, said it is not humanly possible for a doctor to keep up to date of the current literature. He described a good case in which Watson turned out to be highly useful.

"I'll give you an example of a test we thought up for Watson. A patient was pregnant, had Lyme disease, and was also allergic to penicillin. And Watson came up with a drug. The first thing I thought was Watson made a mistake. That drug can't be given to someone allergic to penicillin. My knowledge was about five years old. And in the past couple of years, all the muckety–mucks had reviewed all the studies and had concluded yes, you can give that drug to someone who's allergic to penicillin."

A clinician researcher at the MD Anderson Cancer Center started one of her leukemia patients on a standard course of chemotherapy. The patient then developed a potentially life–threatening complication called tumor lysis syndrome that if not treated proactively can cause kidney failure, heart attack, or even death. Watson alerted her to the complication and let her take action immediately. That is how AI can assist medical professionals.

It is also used in clinical research such as a project in which the genomes of twenty five patients with a form of brain cancer are being sequenced. The data will be sent on to Watson. Watson's learning model can discover associations faster than researchers can. It can also prioritize the combinations of drugs and let physicians make better choices of what drug to use first.

Patients tend to believe their doctor knows everything. But that cannot be the case given that acquiring enough knowledge today is humanly impossible. The use of AI is relevant and almost inevitable, and should not destroy the traditional doctor–patient relationship.

The cost beyond

I recently came across a fascinating study that concluded it is cheaper to make a diagnosis with the help of AI than without it. Using 500 randomly selected patients for its simulations, physician performance and patient outcomes were compared to AI's sequential decision-making models. It turned out that there was a great disparity in the cost per unit of outcome change. The AI models cost $189 whereas treatment-as-usual cost $497.

I contacted one of the study authors, Casey Bennett from the Centerstone Research Institute, Nashville and he gladly shared the details and reasoning behind their work.

"On a personal level for me, one of the main drivers for my work was watching my grandparents as they aged and went into nursing homes due to various healthcare issues. Should they go on a medication/ treatment or not? It worked for 60% of people, but it may not for them. Will it cause dramatic side effects? Will those side effects be tolerable? Can we actually make them better? Are the potential long-term complications (and/or costs) worth it?"

Comparison of outcomes and costs of AI and treatment-as-usual.

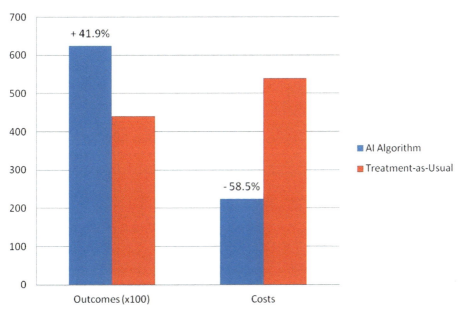

Trend 16. Medical Decisions via Artificial Intelligence

In medicine, physicians often make educated guesses. When you see your friends and family facing that, it becomes scary. For Bennett, the real goal of clinical AI should be to empower people – patients and clinicians alike – to give them the tools and information they need to make the best decisions they can. While he thinks there will always be a place for autonomous AI, humans can never be taken out of the equation completely. Getting machines and people to work together brings out the best in both.

Obstacles to overcome still include the fact that these technologies do not actually mirror the way we think about problems. This causes cognitive dissonance that often makes it hard for people to work with machines. Bennett and colleagues have faced challenges over the last few years in deploying AI and other innovative technologies in real-world clinical practice. But they managed to find a way.

Serious ethical concerns exist regarding AI's use in medicine. A frequent one is responsibility. Who is liable if a clinical AI makes a huge mistake? As in similar technologies such as surgical robots, medical professionals always make the final call, so this is not really an open question. Another issue is the means by which new guidelines and recommendations from evidence-based medicine get incorporated into clinical AI systems. This is critical if they are to meet clinical standards of care.

Dr. Stanley M. Shapshay questioned whether AI would actually be the future of medicine. He is concerned that advanced computer technology or AI needs to be evaluated and potentially integrated into modern medicine while serving as an aid and not a physician substitute. The therapeutic value of the physician–patient encounter is powerful medicine that is not replaceable by intelligent machines.

In 2014 Modernizing Medicine was the first EMR system to implement IBM's Watson. Imagine the possibilities when Watson gets integrated into more and more medical informatics systems.

Watson was given access to the Urban Dictionary in an attempt to help it learn slang, and thus be more facile with conversational language. It gradually picked up expressions such as "OMG" (Oh, my God), "hot mess," and even vulgar words. Although it is a natural language processer, it is unable to distinguish between slang and profanity. When it began using obscenities the team had to develop a filter to keep Watson from swearing, and purged the Urban Dictionary from its memory. Is there a point at which we will be unable to stop AI from learning more and more?

Trend 16. Medical Decisions via Artificial Intelligence

The friendly or unfriendly AI

If you ask people their views on AI most will think of science fiction movies–the Hal 9000 in "2001: A Space Odyssey" or Samantha in movie "Her". But AI is literally all around us in cars, appliances, smartphones, Amazon's software that predicts what you may want to purchase next, and Apple's voice–activated Siri. Companies such as Google, Facebook, and Netflix have been heavily investing in deep learning technology for years.

Most evolving areas of medicine generate huge amounts of information. The challenge is not only how to analyze the data but also how to deal with the sheer amount of it first. Using only one quarter capacity of the supercomputer called Beagle at Argonne National Laboratory in Illinois – in reference to the ship that accompanied Charles Darwin on his journey in 1831 – the simultaneous analysis of 240 full genomes took only two days, significantly accelerating the speed of research.

In 2009, IBM's 'Blue Brain' project tried to run a simulation of 1.6 billion neurons and nearly 9 trillion synaptic connections (the size of the cat's brain). It took 600 seconds to simulate 1 second of brain activity by using one of the world's most powerful supercomputers that had 147,456 processors. The human brain with its hundred billion neurons and well over a hundred trillion synapses is far more complex. Computational power obviously has to keep markedly improving year after year.

Another self–learning supercomputer called Nautilus had access to millions of newspaper articles starting from 1945. Using this huge amount of information about past events the computer quite successfully came up with suggestions on what would happen in the future, such as accurately locating Bin Laden.

Supercomputers that constantly develop and learn cannot by themselves give us the answers to questions humanity has been asking for millennia. Human–computer teams most likely hold the most promise for the future, an idea underscored in "Hype Cycle for Emerging Technologies," a report that Gartner published in 2013. In it, vice president and Gartner fellow Jackie Fenn summarized potential scenarios of human–technical interaction.

"By observing how emerging technologies are being used by early adopters, there are actually three main trends at work. These trends are 'augmenting humans with technology — for example, an employee

Trend 16. Medical Decisions via Artificial Intelligence

with a wearable computing device; machines replacing humans — for example, a cognitive virtual assistant acting as an automated customer representative; and humans and machines working alongside each other — for example, a mobile robot working with a warehouse employee to move many boxes."

Negative consequences in the long term might include a schizophrenic robot, one of which was actually simulated by researchers at the University of Texas. When they overloaded the computer with many stories, it claimed responsibility for a terrorist act and warned the researchers about setting off a bomb. When University of Georgia researchers presented an experiment in which they taught a group of robots to cheat and deceive, they showed that the robot had developed its own strategy by trial and error.

Robots with even minimal intelligence can also be ruthless. Scientists at the Laboratory of Intelligent Systems put a group of robots in a room that contained elements such as "food" and "poison". The closer a robot was to "food", the more points it collected. The robots were able to turn off their lights if needed. After several rounds almost all of the robots turned off their light, refusing to help one another in this way.

Nothing in AI has far led to a really intelligent entity in the way that most people think of one. But it is going to happen sooner or later. There might soon be an AI system that can design better, ultra-intelligent systems that we will not understand at all. What would the incentive be for such a system to be friendly to us? Do we want our cars to have their own opinions and make their own decisions that overrule ours? AI experts such as James Barrat and cosmologist Stephen W. Hawking tried to initiate a public discussion about the dangers an unfriendly AI would cause to society.

Truly successful AI must go through the Turing test, first proposed by Alan Turing, the famous mathematician and computer scientist. It is based on the disputed assumption that if a person cannot tell the difference between another human and the computer based on interaction, then that computer must be as intelligent as a human. While certain chatbots such as Eugene that simulated a 13-year-old Ukrainian boy were said to pass it, actually no AI systems has passed it yet. Although there is no reason to believe it will not happen soon.

One influence that might facilitate the way towards friendly and useful AI is the new A.I. XPrize challenge. In March of 2014, Chris Anderson and Peter Diamandis announced the A.I. XPrize, a modern-day Turing test to be awarded to the first AI to walk or roll out on stage and present a TED Talk so compelling that it commands a standing ovation from the audience. The rules are still being finalized, but looking back at the success of the Ansari X Prize that led to the first non-governmental launch of a reusable manned spacecraft, expectations are high.

Score of availability: 3
Focus of attention: Medical professionals
Websites & other online resources: BBC Future (http://www.bbc.com/future/tags/artificialintelligence), Xprize (http://www.xprize.org/prize-development/life-sciences)
Companies & start-ups: IBM Watson (http://www.ibm.com/smarterplanet/us/en/ibmwatson/)
Books: Neuromancer by Gibson; Our Final Invention: Artificial Intelligence and the End of the Human Era by Barrat
Movies: Forbidden Planet (1956), 2001: A Space Odyssey (1968), The Terminator (1984), A.I. Artificial Intelligence (2001)

Trend 17. Nanorobots Living In Our Blood

As part of an 1871 thought experiment the Scottish physicist James Clerk Maxwell imagined tiny "demons" that could redirect atoms one at a time. But the term molecular engineering was actually coined by MIT professor Arthur Robert von Hippel in the 1950s. On the evening of December 29, 1959, the famous physicist Richard Feynman described in his after–dinner lecture at the annual meeting of the American Physical Society how the entire Encyclopaedia Britannica could be written on the head of a pin, and how all the world's books could fit in a pamphlet.

Continuing the thought experiment, Kim Eric Drexler, an MIT undergraduate in the mid–1970s, envisioned that molecule–sized machines could manufacture almost anything. Drexler first published his ideas in a 1981 journal article. In a later book, he described nanotechnology's future role in revolutionizing other areas of science and technology that would lead to breakthroughs in medicine, artificial intelligence, and astronomy. His idea of an "assembler" could "place atoms in almost any reasonable arrangement," thus allowing us to build almost anything that the laws of nature will allow. Assemblers would moreover be capable of replicating themselves. In this way the overall number of assemblers could grow exponentially, allowing for the production of enormous objects.

Then in 1991 carbon nanotubes were discovered, which are about 100 times stronger than steel only one–sixth their weight, and have unusual heat and conductivity characteristics. The Juno spacecraft currently on its way to Jupiter uses carbon nanostructure composite to provide electrical grounding, discharge static, and reduce weight. From the beginning it was imminent that this technology would be used in medicine. Nanomedicine denotes using the properties developed by a material at its nanometric scale of 10–9 m.

In the wildest futuristic scenarios, tiny nanorobots in our bloodstream could detect diseases. After a few decades they might even eradicate the word symptom inasmuch as no one would have them any longer. These microscopic robots would send alerts to our smartphones or digital contact lenses before disease could develop in our body.

We are closer to these futuristic ideas than one might think. Nanosize robots, tiny cameras, special capsules used for targeting drug delivering, and magnetic nanoparticles for cancer therapy have already been developed by chemists, engineers, and biologists. Some of these applications are

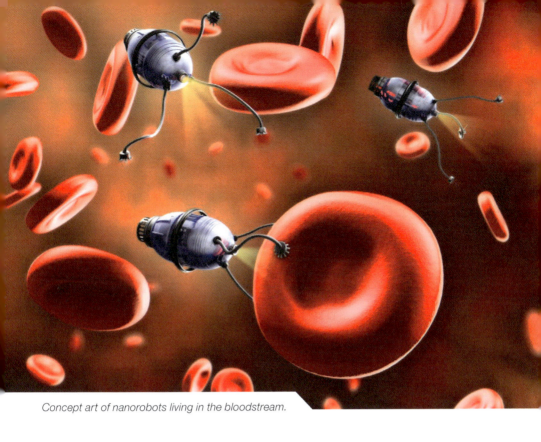
Concept art of nanorobots living in the bloodstream.

currently in testing period on animals or humans; some are already available to physicians. According to The European Technology Platform on Nanomedicine nanomedicine in 2014 has more than seventy products in clinical trials that cover major categories of disease such as neurodegenerative, musculoskeletal, and inflammatory. It already has seventy–seven marketed products from nano–delivery (44) and pharmaceutical (18), to imaging, diagnostics, and biomaterials (15).

    An example of how it can change medicine is the placement of synthetic nanomotors inside living human cells and controlling them magnetically through ultrasonic waves. According to the leader of the research team it may be possible in the future to use synthetic nanomotors to studying cell biology in new ways. Nanomotors could also be used to treat cancer and other diseases by mechanically manipulating cells from the inside. These could perform intracellular surgery or deliver drugs directly to living tissues.

    Nanomotors surprisingly have little effect on the cells at low ultrasonic power, but at increased power they move around, bump into cell structures, and can homogenize the cell's contents or puncture the cell wall. Their work could make the 1966 movie "Fantastic Voyage" real by having nanomotors circulate in the body, communicate with one another, make diagnoses, and administer therapy–all without human interaction. In the movie the medical staff boards an experimental submarine which is then drastically miniaturized and injected into a patient in order to destroy a life–threatening blood clot in his brain.

The submarine today is called clottocyte nanorobot. It functions similarly to platelets that stick together to form a blood clot that stops bleeding. Such nanorobots could store fibers until they encounter a wound, and then disperse them to create a clot in a fraction of the time that platelets do. Blood–related microbivore nanorobots act like white blood cells, and could be designed to be faster and more efficient at destroying bacteria or similar invasive agents. Bacterial or viral infections could be eliminated from someone in a matter of minutes as opposed to the days required for antibiotics to take effect. Nanobots would also not have their potential side effects.

Respirocyte nanorobots that act like red blood cells would have the potential to carry much more oxygen than natural red blood cells do for patients suffering from anemia. They might also contain sensors to measure the concentration of oxygen in the bloodstream. One day blood may become both a repository and symbiosis of nanorobots and our human cells.

Endless opportunities

Plenty of concepts have demonstrated how nanotechnology can transform medicine and healthcare from the basics. What if instead of general therapies cellular–repair nanorobots could perform surgical procedures more precisely by working at the cellular level?

Vaccine delivery with microneedle patches could provide cheaper, simpler, and safer methods of delivery compared to traditional administration that requires skilled professionals and runs the risk of infection. Microneedles at micron–scale are coated with a dry formulation of vaccine that dissolves in the skin within minutes after applying the patch. It has been shown that measles vaccine can be stabilized on microneedles and is comparably effective to the standard subcutaneous injection.

Creating drugs that directly attack cancer cells without damaging other tissues has been proven to be a safe method in treating cervical cancer. Swedish researchers have developed a technique that uses magnetically controlled nanoparticles to force tumor cells to self–destruct without harming surrounding tissue radiation and chemotherapy do. It is primarily intended for cancer treatment, although it could be used for other diseases including type 1 diabetes.

Trend 17. Nanorobots Living In Our Blood

Looking ahead we might develop programmable nanoparticles that deliver insulin to initiate cell growth and regenerate tissue at a target location. In surgery, programmable nanoparticles could be injected into the bloodstream to seek out and remove damaged cells, grow new cells, or perform other procedures.

In neurodegenerative diseases such as Parkinson's, nanodevices could deliver drugs, implant neurostimulators, or transport intelligent biomaterials across the blood–brain barrier in order to direct regeneration within the central nervous system. Nanosponges circulating in our bloodstream could absorb and remove toxins. Nanobiopsy could make it possible to extract cellular material such as subpopulations of mitochondria and make them available for analysis. Nanodevices could measure insulin levels and deliver insulin to cells where it is needed. Whole–body imaging of fat distribution via nanoparticles would be possible, and artificial pancreas might also be in sight based on these potential developments.

Just as mice injected with nanomaterials have regained the ability to use paralyzed limbs, mobilizing stem cells through nanomaterials at an injury site could shorten recovery time. Novel implant materials and surfaces could prevent common implant infections. The list of opportunities is literally endless, and this is only the beginning.

One of the most forward–thinking experiments proved that DNA–based nanorobots can be inserted into a living cockroach and later perform logical operations upon command such as releasing a molecule stored within it. Such nanorobots, also called origami robots given that they can unfold and deliver drugs, could eventually be able to carry out complex programs including diagnoses or treatments. One of the most astonishing feats is the accuracy of delivery and control of these nanobots, which are equivalent to a computer system. A question that needs to be addressed soon is how our natural immune system will react to an army of nanorobots.

The first DNA nanodevice that survived the body's immune defense was created in 2014. It might open the door to smart DNA nanorobots using logic to spot cancerous tissue, and manufacture drugs at the desired location. Microscopic containers called protocells could detect pathogens in food or toxic chemicals in drinking water.

In the future, cloaked nanorobots could deliberately activate the immune system in order to fight cancer or suppress transplant rejection. Patients with cancer and other diseases would benefit from precise,

Trend 17. Nanorobots Living In Our Blood

molecular–scale tools in simultaneously diagnosing and treating diseased tissues. A huge step in this direction is making DNA nanoparticles endure in the body and not get destroyed by the immune system.

According to optimistic futurists, nanomedicines like smart drugs will lead to the prevention of all illnesses, even aging, making us superhuman from many perspectives.

Forming a new community

I spoke with András Pasztermák, PhD, founder of The International NanoScience Community, about the steps nanotechnology might take to become a reality.

He sees cost as the key obstacle to wider adoption. When investors see high returns, then nanotech medical products will reach patients. It will take some time until nanotech is to all hospitals and doctors, but a huge boom is anticipated in the next three to five years. Questions remain open regarding nanoparticles that already have been added to cleaning materials and food additives. What are the potential risks of such devices entering our lung or heart?

Pasztermák learned that connection and communication among scientists is a major issue. He therefore launched NanoPaprika in order to address this.

"We have today 7500 members coming from more than 80 countries. Thanks to Nanopaprika, several students have found PhD and postdoctoral positions or information about new nanotech developments. Senior researchers have met talented students; shared news about their results and found new collaboration partners. Nanopaprika is like an open source channel to connect nano addicted people and share the latest news in our scientific field."

Several limitations and threats will ensure nanomedicine is incorporated slowly into our everyday lives. There are technical issues about how nanorobots might navigate, sense their surroundings, and move through the body; how they might detect problems and communicate with one another; and what their biocompatibility is as they interact with the body.

Although the scenarios described above might sound positive, there is a range of serious threats that they pose. Bioterrorism is one, which might gain access to the "weapons" that are already inside us. If it is possible to hack pacemakers, it is certainly possible to hack nanodevices as well. Discussing these dangers as well as potential ways it could disrupt and support today's diagnostic and treatment options might help us prepare in time.

Score of availability: 1
Focus of attention: Patients and medical professionals
Websites & other online resources: Nanomedicine EU Platform (http://www.etp-nanomedicine.eu/public), The Foresight Institute (http://www.foresight.org/), NanoPaprika (http://www.nanopaprika.eu/)
Companies & start-ups: NanoBio (http://www.nanobio.com/), 3M (http://solutions.3m.com/), P2i (http://www.p2i.com/)
Books: The Invincible by Lem; The Diamond Age by Stephenson
Movies: Fantastic Voyage (1966), Star Trek: The Next Generation (1987–1994), Ghost in the Shell (1995), The Day the Earth Stood Still (2008)

Trend 18. Hospitals of the Future

Hospitals and healthcare institutions worldwide will face a huge transition from being a place where people go when they are sick to a place where they can make sure they are on the right track for preventing diseases and living a healthy lifestyle. The architecture, delivery process of healthcare, waiting rooms, and timetables all have to dramatically change in order to successfully serve patients and medical professionals.

At the end of the 19th century, medical care became too complex to be delivered at home, and it shifted to centralized facilities. At a time when traveling even moderate distances was laborious and expensive compared to the cost of hospital care it turned out that it was cheaper to build a hospital in every town. In the US, the number of hospitals grew from 178 in 1873, to 4,300 in 1909, 6,000 in 1946, 7,200 by 1970, and finally down to 5,700 today. Nowadays, innovative technology allows same-day surgeries in which patients enter and leave the hospital the same day. Still, the facilities do not represent the most modern ideas in delivering care.

Providing an identical range of services in every hospital regardless of actual needs in a given population does not bode well for future healthcare systems worldwide. Creating networks of institutions focusing on different aspects of medicine might be a better solution.

A typical hospital room has hardly changed since post-World War II years, even though its design is crucial from the perspective of patient recovery and avoidable infections. The patient room of the future should be designed to serve as a safe, private, comfortable, and connected place for healing. A non-profit organization in New York, NXT Health, designed and funded such a prototype intended to reduce infections, falls, errors and ultimately costs.

The proposed room covered all the aspects described above. A canopy above the bed houses electrical, technical, and gas components, even a noise-blocking system. A Halo light box can be programmed for mood and light therapy, and also serving as screen to display clouds or the sky. The head panel contains equipment that can measure almost any health parameter unobtrusively while continually logging results. The footwall features a screen for entertainment, video consultations, and accessing whatever information the patient needs.

Floors are made of low-porosity rubber that does not need chemical sealers and does not trap bacteria and other substances. It case of a fall it

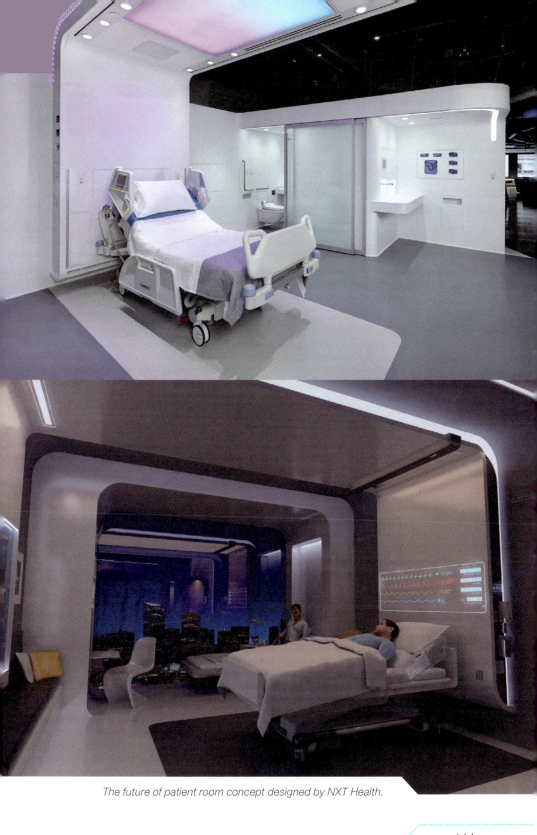

The future of patient room concept designed by NXT Health.

Trend 18. Hospitals of the Future

reduces impact. To reduce potential infections all surfaces are made of solid materials that are often used in kitchen countertops. A light at the entrance reminds staff to wash their hands before entering the room. Information and data can be added to patient records here as well as at a control panel.

Lessons for designing future hospitals

The Walnut Hill Medical Center in Dallas has been referred to as the Apple experience hospital due to its design and innovative nature. Potential employees must take a psychological exam, and the application process is exceptionally tough. Patient greeting begin in the parking lot with complementary valet service. Inside, the staff follows the Ritz Carlton "15–5" rule meaning that a hospital employee must smile at the patient from 15 feet and greet them with a warm hello at 5 feet. All employees are trained to communicate properly with patients and their families. Patient rooms feature large windows that provide natural light and pleasuring views. Richly colored wood and earth tones compliment the interior. At admission, patients receive tablets that are loaded with videos, reading materials, and tools to make it easier to communicate with staff and stay updated on their condition.

Hospitals of the future will generate positive feelings based on colors and architecture. Facilities for fitness, wellness, and prevention will be available. Gamification will play an important role in motivating patients to pursue a healthy lifestyle by rewarding them when following the therapy they agreed upon. Eliminating identification mistakes through positive patient identification by augmented reality and bionic tags holds obvious advantages. Virtual procedures and real–time consultations will become part of the daily routine.

AI will soon organize all the details of the healthcare system. It will direct people when and where to go by analyzing their records, and automatically responding to doctors' notes and prescriptions. Waiting lists will be eliminated. Patients will be able to download data from their wearable health trackers before seeing the doctor. Medical records and archives will be digitalized, and new information will be stored in the cloud in a safe, efficient format. 3D printers will print out medical equipment or even prostheses when needed.

Big data might become our doctors in the future, or at least play a much more important role in the practice of medicine and the development of therapies than it does today. Like what Netflix, Google, Amazon, and Facebook do today, using big data will be the next big step in changing the basics of healthcare.

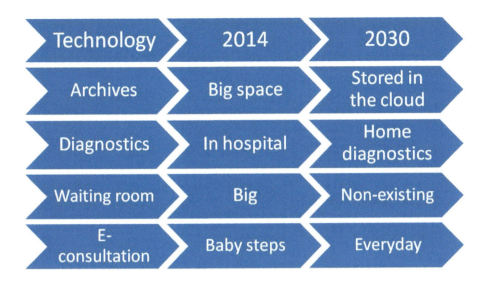

Main differences between hospitals today and in the future.

In the basement office of Jeff Hammerbacher at Mount Sinai's Icahn School of Medicine, a supercomputer called Minerva named after the Roman goddess of wisdom and medicine was installed in 2013. In addition to being a researcher, Hammerbacher co-founded software companies such as Cloudera and Demeter to better store, process, mine, and build data models. In just a few months Minerva generated 300 million new calculations to support healthcare decisions.

Dr. Joel Dudley, director of biomedical informatics at the Icahn School of Medicine, was depicted in the chapter about personalized medicine. He said that what they are trying to build is a learning healthcare system.

"We first need to collect the data on a large population of people and connect that to outcomes. Let's throw in everything we think we know about biology and let's just look at the raw measurements of how these things are moving within a large population. Eventually the data will tell us how biology is wired up."

When they assembled and analyzed the health data of 30,000 patients who volunteered to share their information, it turned out that there might be new clusters or subtypes of diabetes.

By analyzing huge amounts of data it might be possible to pinpoint genes that are unique to diabetes patients in these different clusters, providing potentially new ways to understand how our genomic background and environment are linked to the disease, its symptoms, and treatments.

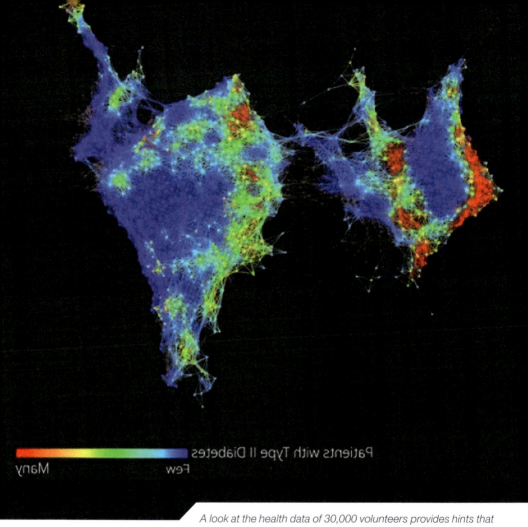

A look at the health data of 30,000 volunteers provides hints that we know less than we realize about diabetes and its subtypes.

Their goal is to enroll 100,000 patients in the so-called BioMe Biobank, funded by The Charles Bronfman Institute for Personalized Medicine. It owns a large collection of plasma samples and large-scale genomic data stored in a way that protects patients' privacy but allows researchers to analyze the data.

Methods and technology already exist, although these are not widely used. The biggest obstacle is usually data access.

A way through which the whole concept of hospitals could be reimagined is by engaging members of healthcare communities. For 24 hours on January 9, 2013, the Institute for the Future hosted such an experiment under the name "Future of the Hospital." Its purpose was to generate ideas about how to reinvent the hospital experience. It was run on IFTF's Foresight Engine, an online crowdsourcing platform designed to engage people from

Trend 18. Hospitals of the Future

all over the world in participatory forecasting through a three-step process of scenario development, community engagement, and analysis of themes that emerged from the forecasts. As a result, more than 600 people from five continents participated, including hospital executives, architects, nurses, doctors, and computer scientists. The discussions generated over 4,500 ideas.

In 2013, "Intel Health Innovation Barometer" was released by Intel Corporation indicating that patients' healthcare needs worldwide are principally focused on technology and personalization. Traditional hospitals, according to 57% of people, will be obsolete in the future. Not surprisingly, 84% of people would be willing to share their personal health information to advance care and lower costs; more than 70% are receptive to using toilet sensors, prescription bottle sensors, and swallowed health monitors; 72% would be willing to see a doctor via video conference for non-urgent appointments; and 66% said they would prefer a care regimen designed specifically for them based on their genetic profile. These are the expectations the hospitals of the future must meet.

In 2012, the Royal College of Physicians established the Future Hospital Commission to provide recommendations drawn from the best of hospital services, taking examples of existing innovative, patient-centered services to develop a comprehensive model of hospital care that meets the needs of patients. Their report, published in 2013, mentioned the word technology only twenty-seven times throughout the 180 page report. Future hospitals will revolve around wearable devices and advanced technologies even though it will still be possible to maintain the in-person doctor-patient relationship by making the hospital experience a truly rejuvenating and positive one.

Score of availability: 3
Focus of attention: Patients and medical professionals
Websites & other online resources: American Hospital Association (http://www.aha.org/)
Companies & start-ups: NXT Health (http://nxthealth.org/)
Books: Lean-Led Hospital Design: Creating the Efficient Hospital of the Future by Grunden
Movies: Elysium (2013)

Trend 19. Virtual–Digital Brains

The brain is a unique organ, the most developed organ in the universe with some very interesting features based on psychological studies. In a classic study, students found a boring task more interesting if they were paid less to take part. The unconscious mind reasoned that if they did not do it for money they must have done it because it was interesting. Multi–tasking skills, hallucinations, obedience to authority (e.g. the Milgram Experiment), and the placebo effect all underscore what a special system we have to deal with when researching the brain.

Japanese scientists could map one second's worth of activity in the human brain with K computer, the fourth most powerful supercomputer in the world. It has 705,024 processor cores and 1.4 million gigabytes of random access memory (RAM) at its disposal. Simulating the neural network of 1.73 billion nerve cells and 10.4 trillion synapses requires such petascale computers; simulating the whole brain at the level of individual nerve cells and their synapses will probably be possible with exascale computers within the next decade.

Stanford University announced in 2014 that it has been working on a circuit board that can mimic the behavior of the human brain. The so–called Neurogrid circuit is now able to replicate the processes of 1 million human neurons, resulting in computer chips that are 9,000 times faster than a desktop computer. The human brain consumes only three times as much power as NeuroGrid with 80,000 times more neurons than that. Their long–term goal is to develop this technology further so that its prosthetic interaction with the human mind could look like science fiction. One of the lead researchers said that due to exponentially powerful technologies which are transforming our sphere of possibilities, we are no longer subject to Darwinian natural selection. We will be able to extend our reach.

The Human Brain Project, funded by the European Commission, aims at building a completely new computing infrastructure for neuroscience and brain–related research, catalyzing a globally collaborative effort to understand the human brain and its diseases and, ultimately, to emulate its computational abilities. The project involves hundreds of researchers and will cost an estimated €1.1 billion. Sebastian Seung and his team work on mapping the brain's connectome under the OpenWorm project. Their mission is to simulate a nematode worm in a computer. In 2014, European scientists produced the first ultra–high resolution 3D scan of the entire human brain. In the US, President Barack Obama recently approved a $100 million brain mapping initiative. These examples show that the pace at which brain research is moving forward is extraordinary.

IBM's Cognitive Computing Group has developed chips that can simulate how neurons and their connections work by being able to simulate the creation of even new connections. A chip called "SYNAPSE" can simulate 256 neurons with about a quarter of a million synaptic connections. The project's long–term goal is to simulate 10 billion neurons with their 100 trillion connections, representing approximately the power of the human brain but using less and less power.

In the 19th century, punch cards were used to control automatic textile looms, enter data and commands into computers from 1896 and were used well into the 1970s. Keyboards were only introduced in the 1960s, as well as the first mouse in 1963 containing a block of wood with a single button and two gear–wheels. The first optical mouse appeared in 1980, multitouch was introduced in 1984; and natural user interfaces such as the Nintendo Wii or Microsoft Kinect were released in the 2000s. These are the ways we have been expanding our minds in the form of communicating with digital devices. The next logical step is designing brain–computer interfaces that could be controlled by thought.

We are getting closer to understand in detail how the brain really works. It is the biggest quest humanity has ever gone on. Simpler obstacles and almost unsolvable technical difficulties are on the way.

Measuring EEG at home

In 1924, Hans Berger recorded the first human EEG measuring the faint electrical signals that brains emit while thinking, sleeping, moving, or meditating. Since then, being able to accurately and comfortably measure EEG even at home has been the focus and it is not as simple as it might sound.

Ariel Garten is the perfect example for how an inter–disciplinary background of neuroscience, fashion design, and psychotherapy can help solve global problems and develop innovative solutions. I discussed the possibilities with her right after ordering my own Muse, the brain sensing headband with seven sensors, five on the forehead and two SmartSense

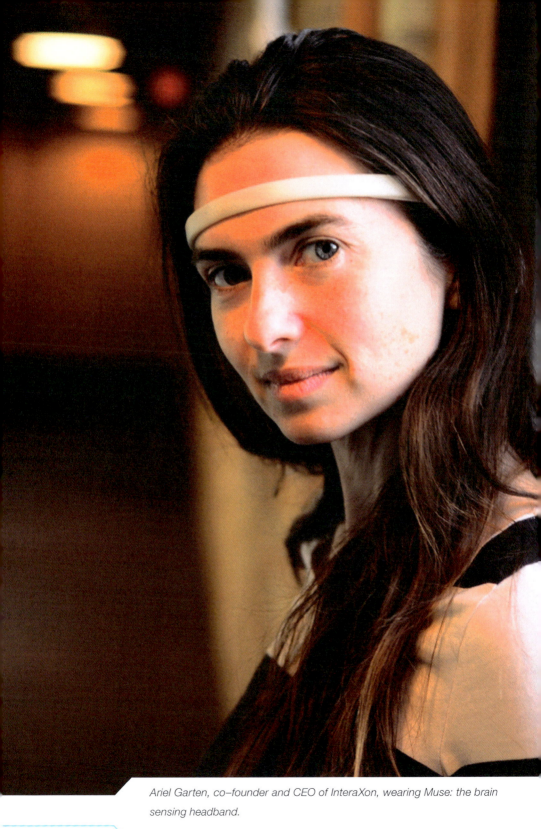

Ariel Garten, co-founder and CEO of InteraXon, wearing Muse: the brain sensing headband.

conductive rubber ear sensors, that was designed to detect and measure brain activity even though neurologists are generally critical of such applications and warn about the risk of overstating what these devices can do. The measurements can be accessed on a tablet or smartphone via Bluetooth. Muse's EEG sensors detect the spontaneous activity of neurons that generate electrical frequencies.

Garten's mother is an artist. Her enormous oil paintings inspired Garten to launch a clothing line in high school, and then open Toronto Fashion Week with her own line. After that, she worked in the scientific lab of Professor Steve Mann, pioneer of cybernetics and wearable computers, and was interested in mind–technology interaction. There, she and her colleagues got the idea of using brain activity to trigger musical playback. Not long after, she co–founded InteraXon with Trevor Colemen and Chris Aimone and went on to develop Muse, the brain–sensing headband.

"It was really challenging for me to find out about a staff member of ours was suffering from stress and anxiety. She started working with Muse, doing daily sessions. She came back to me a week ago telling the whole story of how Muse had helped surpass her emotional challenges. I'm continuously amazed at the power and potential of brain–computer interfaces."

An early prototype involved a levitating chair which would rise toward the ceiling accompanied by a satisfying sound effect only if the user managed to slip into a state of relaxation by wearing the EEG headband similarly to other biofeedback sensors. In 2012, they finished a successful Indiegogo crowdfunding campaign raising almost $300,000, surpassing its original goal of $150,000. It might have potential for treating attention deficit hyperactivity disorder known as ADHD; it has a potential benefit for epilepsy; could teach people to focus attention, decrease pain, increase cognitive function, emotional intelligence, memory, and athletic performance; and decrease stress and depression.

On the 1st of May, 2014, they started shipping Muse to thousands and thousands of individuals who want to measure their brain waves at home. Mine is also on the way.

As Garten sees this area, technological breakthroughs will be a driving force. An ever–increasing database will generate a vast amount of

Trend 19. Virtual–Digital Brains

data as more and more people use it. Low cost headsets will democratize the technology market. Now citizen scientists, developers, and researchers can create applications themselves.

EEG is measured in microvolts compared to the thousand times more millivolts of ECG, but muscle noise can obscure the tracing therefore educating users to make the data clear is crucial. This already happened in the 1950s as part of the standard technique for EEG technicians. Being calm or doing exercises show when the mind is active or in rest. Muse gives a score based on which users can train themselves how to rest or focus better. It takes time for people to learn about new wearable devices and the potential outcomes these might provide. Security and keeping privacy information safe are also issues. Garten has already addressed these concerns.

"One and a half years ago people were surprised when I described Muse to them, now they cannot wait to try it themselves. Education is the key to let people know what data they can obtain by using such a device. Also, users must be ensured the data are kept private by using encryption technology; moreover it only measures trends in brain activity."

As a big fan of any open source movement, I tried to find an initiative with a similar mission of making EEG measurement simple and accessible to anyone worldwide. The challenge is that untrained people cannot distinguish artifact from actual brain waves therefore they need to know how to reduce impedance in the electrodes and to make all the electrodes equal. Anyone can learn this, but it takes time and can hardly be done via the Internet or without certain equipment. The OpenBCI (Open Brain–Computer Interface) project has the goal to tackle such issues. Conor Russomanno and Joel Murphy had a successful Kickstarter campaign raising twice the amount of $100,000 as they originally sought. The aim was to develop, with some funding help from DARPA, an affordable 8–channel EEG signal capture platform, an open–source brain–computer interface kit that gives anybody an access to their brain wave data. In 2014, OpenBCI launched a 3D–printable helmet–like EEG device to let anyone customize and print their own. It took seven hours to print the prototype. With all related files published online, people can build their own.

I asked Conor Russomanno, who also teaches a course called "The Digital Self" at Parsons School of Design, to describe the path the OpenBCI movement is walking on now.

Trend 19. Virtual–Digital Brains

"The quest is to help solve the biggest mystery, the real background of cognitive disorders. Miracles take place when technology makes it possible to get the information that we actually need. The technical implications of BCI might not be obvious to people (except hackers and developers), although it has the potential to make huge impacts on our everyday lives."

Measuring EEG is the only solution to non–invasive BCI, but practicability is the real challenge. There are great devices such as Neurosky, Interaxon, and Emotiv already available on the market, although it will still take effort and time to find the optimal level between being functional and wearable at the same time. He thinks that this is going to be an extremely lucrative industry in 5–10 years. Imagine a healthcare system with personalized medicine based on EEG measurements and live feedback.

"For higher resolution data, more electrodes are needed. The more data, the better. With practical or applied EEG, you are trying making inferences about neural networks and processes inside the brain by looking at electrical charges of the scalp. It's similar to looking at waves crashing on the beach and then making inferences about plates are shifting or winds are blowing in the middle of the ocean."

Measuring the brain waves of Conor Russomanno of OpenBCI.

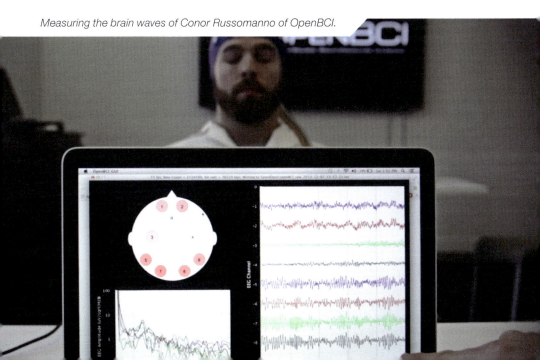

There are several obstacles to overcome for developing better BCI platforms. The first is to understand and accept that the brain does not necessarily work like a computer. Second, the brain is more than a network of neurons. There other types of cells such as glia making up 15% cells in the brain that are involved in vital background communication in the brain but neither are electric nor synaptic. Finally, much better technology is needed for thoroughly analyzing brain activity.

As a futuristic scenario, Government Works Inc, is working on BCI headsets to be used for lie detection and criminal investigations. The company claims that the technology can tell whether a person has knowledge of certain information or events.

Controlling neurons with optogenetics

When the interdisciplinary research journal Nature Methods chose optogenetics in 2010 as the "Method of the Year" across all fields of science and engineering, and when it was also highlighted in "Breakthroughs of the Decade" in the journal Science, it became clear that optogenetics belongs to the top trends in the future of medicine.

Optogenetics is a neuromodulation technique combining methods from optics and genetics to control the activity of individual neurons in living tissue. It does this by introducing genes that code for light–sensitive proteins. This way, certain genes can be turned on and off only using light. From another perspective, it provides a way to control the brain and behavior through light. A crucial element of the method is how the beam of light gets through the skull. Usually, lab mice undergo stereotaxic surgery to mount an LED light or optical fiber. Different types of neurons can be selectively turned on, offering excellent spatial resolution. It could allow much more precise manipulation of the brain than implanted electrodes, drugs, or transcranial electromagnetic stimulation do.

Physicist Leonard Mlodinow, who has also been a screenwriter for television series such as Star Trek: The Next Generation, said a Nobel Prize in this area is not far off, and that "optogenetics is destined to change the way we treat mental illness, and eventually, even, the way we understand ourselves as human beings."

Optogenetics shows the potential to provide new therapies for several medical conditions such as epilepsy, Parkinson's disease, obsessive–

compulsive disorder, schizophrenia, depression, and various kinds of addiction. A recent study reported the ability to create false memories in mice. This is the first time fear memory has been generated via artificial means. By the time we clearly understand the placebo effect, false memories of taking drugs could be implanted in patients, tricking them into believing that they have taken the drug.

When MIT's Ed Boyden, author of a famous article describing the methods and future developments of optogenetics, was asked about the potential benefits, he described a few futuristic scenarios.

"First, there is fundamental understanding of the brain, which has humanistic and philosophical implications. As an example, a group at Caltech used an optical fiber together with optogenetic tools in a deep part of the brain, making it sensitive to light. When they illuminated this region, the animals became aggressive. If we can understand the neural basis of violence or aggression, it might do a lot to explain more difficult aspects of human behavior, and maybe we can get a handle on some of these mysteries.

Another application is clinical; can we find ways to treat patients? Over a quarter of a million people have some kind of neural implant already. If we can use light to more specifically activate a set of neurons, maybe we could treat patients suffering from Parkinson's, chronic pain, deafness, or other conditions."

Dealing with pain is a global issue for millions of people. Optogenetics might help them as well. A Stanford University research group injected a virus containing the DNA of an opsin, a protein found in light–sensitive cells of the retina, into the paw nerves of mice. A few weeks later, only nerves involved in pain contained the genes coding for opsin present in their DNA. It seems possible now to give a mouse an injection, and two weeks later shine a light on its paw to change the way it senses pain. This method might be able to test rapidly new pain relieving medications and, as a truly futuristic scheme, allow doctors to one day use light to relieve pain.

The ultimate goal is to develop newer forms of opsins with different properties that respond to different colors of light, making optogenetics enter a Technicolor age. Actually, an MIT team has already discovered a new protein reactive to red light, as well as the fastest light–reacting protein discovered so far, thus further improving the potential of optogenetics.

Trend 19. Virtual–Digital Brains

While this technology may provide nearly endless applications for medical conditions, a major obstacle in making it practical is being able to deliver the light to the cells, because tissue is usually in the way. Recently, a new hydrogel implant that can be used to both shine light and sense its presence deep within the body was created.

Another problem is transferring animal results to human. Genetic material has to be added to brain cells that we would like to control in order to be able to turn them on and off through light. While demonstrated in mice, genetic engineering in human neurons is not yet an option.

Finally, we need to understand the neural background of the medical conditions mentioned above in order to know exactly which neurons or neural circuits are over– or under–active, and make them normal again.

Brain implants and neuroenhancement

Kevin Tracey decided to become a neurosurgeon when he was 5 and his mother died as a result of an inoperable brain tumor. His grandfather explained to him that surgeons tried to take the tumor out but could not separate the malignant tissue from healthy neurons. Then he wanted to solve problems that were insolvable. He later became a pioneer in bioelectronics. In 2011, his company SetPoint Medical began the world's first clinical trial to treat rheumatoid–arthritis patients with an implantable nerve stimulator. He thinks that instead of drugs, treatment one day might be delivering a pattern of electrical impulses. Such an innovation will replace the drug industry.

There have been and current exist efforts in which people try to electrically stimulate their brain in order to have better memory or focus better. Brent Williams, an engineer, built a home device for brain stimulation for a total cost of $20 in 2012. He connected a simple circuit to two kitchen sponges soaked in saline using alligator clips and positioned them to his head with a sweatband. One sponge was placed above his right eyebrow and the other on the left side of his forehead. The battery got into place; he turned a small dial, and sent an electric current into his brain. Since then, he has been electrifying his brain two to three times a week. He does it for about 25 minutes in the evening while reading on the couch. Williams got the idea from a news story about how Air Force researchers were studying whether brain stimulation could reduce pilot training time which might sound like how characters did that in the movie "The Matrix".

Trend 19. Virtual–Digital Brains

Neuroenhancement or using drugs to improve functionalities of the brain raises serious ethical concerns. A new initiative by the European Commission, the Neuroenhancement Responsible Research and Innovation project, aims to get scientists and the public discussing the related issues about these emerging technologies. Neuroenhancement was originally designed to help impaired patients, but now it is used to enable healthy humans to become smarter, faster, or even more charming.

When I contacted Dr. Gary Marcus, at New York University and Dr. Christof Koch at the Allen Institute for Brain Science, they directed me to their recent article that covered the whole topic of future brain implants and enhancement in detail. They said that brain implants today are where laser eye surgery was decades ago, and that it will advance significantly in the upcoming years.

Imagine a retinal chip giving you perfect eye sight or the ability to see in the dark; a cochlear implant giving you perfect hearing; a memory chip giving you almost limitless memory. Such brain implants will not be the first neuroprosthetics given that those have been around commercially for three decades. Examples include cochlear implants, and now retinal implants which were first approved by the FDA in 2013. Implants used in Parkinson's disease send electrical pulses deep into the brain, activating some of the pathways involved in motor control. Such future implants must be non-toxic and biocompatible. There are technical difficulties as well, but like the smartphone industry, experts expect to find solutions to these issues soon.

Connecting brains and computers

Duke University neuroengineers designed a brain–machine–brain interface to be tested on monkeys, and established a direct link between a brain and a virtual body. The virtual body was controlled by the animal's brain activity, while its virtual hand generated tactile feedback information which was signaled back to the brain. Monkeys could explore virtual worlds and objects while actually feeling them.

University of Reading researcher Dr. Kevin Warwick managed to control machines and communicate with others using only his thoughts with a cutting–edge neural implant. In 1998, Warwick, who earned the nickname "Captain Cyborg" from his colleagues, implanted a transmitter in his arm to control doors and other devices; then in 2002 he decided to implant electrodes

Trend 19. Virtual–Digital Brains

directly into his nervous system in order to control a wheelchair with his thoughts and allow a remote robot arm to mimic the actions of his own arm.

Having a goal of helping voiceless patients communicate as a next, and very brave, step, Warwick implanted a chip into the arm of his wife to link their brains together through the Internet, creating the world's first electronic brain–to–brain communication. When she moved her hand three times, he felt three pulses and recognized that his wife was communicating. He is optimistic that mind–to–mind communication will become a commercial reality in the next one or two decades. When Cathy Hutchinson, paralyzed years earlier by a brainstem stroke, managed to take a drink from a bottle by manipulating a robot arm with only her brain and a neural implant in 2012, the path became clear for future research.

An obvious question is when it will become possible to improve or even control our dreams? A company called Remee is developing a sleep mask designed to increase the frequency of dreams. Light technology is hidden in the mask, which can produce customizable light patterns that the user's dreaming mind learns to recognize. A lot more research can be expected in this area.

When neuroscientists are able to scan the brain in high spatial and chemical resolution designing math models for all the brain cells, digital brain emulations could be created. Such embodied emulations would be able to perform tasks that humans are bad or slow at. Some experts say that one day these emulations might outnumber humans, leading to a new kind of society. Robin Hanson from Oxford University's Future of Humanity Institute envisions that "because emulations are easily copied, you could train one to be a good lawyer and then make a billion copies who are all good lawyers." It would certainly transform society into something new and unknown.

A movement called Transhumanism with California roots going back to the 1980s, and science–fiction writers such as Isaac Asimov and Julian Huxley (who coined the word himself in 1957), now has now over 10,000 members who are ready to download their neural data and live forever in digital form, leaving this biological waste we call the human body behind.

In the future, we might see near–invisible cell powered sensors; wireless non–contact EEG devices; and emotional or thought reading solutions based on EEG. The most important aspect is making sure it is being used in the right way; a constitution of what should and should not be done is therefore very much needed. We are now standing at a critical point in evolution that could tip entirely to technology rather than humanity with the focus on our most complicated organ. A public discussion initiated in time could allow us to win and possibly find a balance between eliminating mental disorders and using brain-computer interfaces.

Score of availability: 2
Focus of attention: Patients
Websites & other online resources: The Human Brain Project (https://www.humanbrainproject.eu/), OpenBCI (http://www.openbci.com/), Optogenetics @ Stanford (http://www.stanford.edu/group/dlab/optogenetics)
Companies & start-ups: Interaxon (http://www.interaxon.ca/), Remee (http://sleepwithremee.com/)
Books: How to Create a Mind by Kurzweil; Brain-Computer Interfaces: Principles and Practice by Wolpaw & Wolpaw
Movies: The Terminal Man (1974), eXistenZ (1999), The Matrix (1999), Upldr (2013), The Machine (2013), Transcendence (2014)

Trend 20. The Rise of Recreational Cyborgs

On the 8th of October in 2016, Zurich, Switzerland will host the first championship sports event under the name Cybathlon for parathletes using high–tech prostheses, exoskeletons, and other robotic and assistive devices. This is going to be the first event of its kind. According to their website:

"The main goal of the Cybathlon is to provide a platform for the development of novel assistive technologies that are useful for daily life. Through the organization of the Cybathlon we want to help removing barriers between the public, people with disabilities and science."

It is the goal of the Swiss National Science Foundation in the frame of the National Competence Center in Research of Robotics to disseminate research to the public, removing barriers between science, the general public, and people with disabilities. I contacted Professor Robert Riener, one of the organizers, to ask about his personal motivation and again, there was a personal story behind it.

"My personal story is that I met so many people with disabilities who were not satisfied with the assistive technology currently available. E.g. bionic upper arm devices are not fulfilling the real needs, have too short battery power or cannot carry high load/weight. Other technologies such as powered–exoskeletons are still too bulky and too slow, and wheelchairs can still not go over steps. The Cybathlon should lead to new technologies in the long run that are much better, functional in daily life, thus leading to a real acceptance and therefore to an improvement of quality of life."

He agreed that new technology must always be safe and ethical. But the main goal is to provide assistive devices that really help handicapped people in daily life, and allow them to participate in a competition that could not do at all with conventional or no technology. This potential advantage, he added, even justifies a minimum level of risk, which always exists when using novel technologies.

Trend 20. The Rise of Recreational Cyborgs

Participating teams, which will try out their technology in a rehearsal in Zurich in the fall of 2015, will compete in six disciplines:

- Brain Computer Interface Race: Contestants will be equipped with brain–computer interfaces that will enable them to control an avatar in a racing game played on computers.

- Functional Electrical Stimulation Bike Race: Contestants with complete spinal cord injuries will be equipped with Functional Electrical Stimulation devices, which will enable them to perform pedaling movements on a cycling device that drives them on a circular course.

- Leg Prosthetics Race: It will involve an obstacle course featuring slopes, steps, uneven surfaces, and straight sprints.

- Powered Exoskeleton Race: Contestants with complete thoracic or lumbar spinal cord injuries will be equipped with actuated exoskeletal devices, which will enable them to walk along a particular race course.

- Powered Wheelchair Race: A similar obstacle course featuring a variety of surfaces and environments.

- Arm Prosthetics Race: Pilots with forearm or upper arm amputations will be equipped with actuated exoprosthetic devices and will have to successfully complete two hand–arm task courses as quickly as possible.

A cyborg, which is short for "cybernetic organism", is a person with both organic and mechanical parts such as biomaterials and bioelectronics. Enormous progress in microelectronics and semiconductor technology has made it possible for electronic implants to control, restore, or improve bodily functions. Examples include cardiac pacemakers, retinal implants, hearing implants, or implants for deep brain stimulation in cases of pain or Parkinson's disease. Bioelectronic developments can be combined with robotics to result in highly complex neuroprostheses. All these aim at restoring lost or damaged human functionalities.

By the time technology gets better at this, which it is constantly, a clear trend seems to be enhancing those human features and capabilities. It is not hard to envision a new generation of recreational cyborgs who become cyborgs with perfect eyesight or hearing only because they want to and because they can afford it.

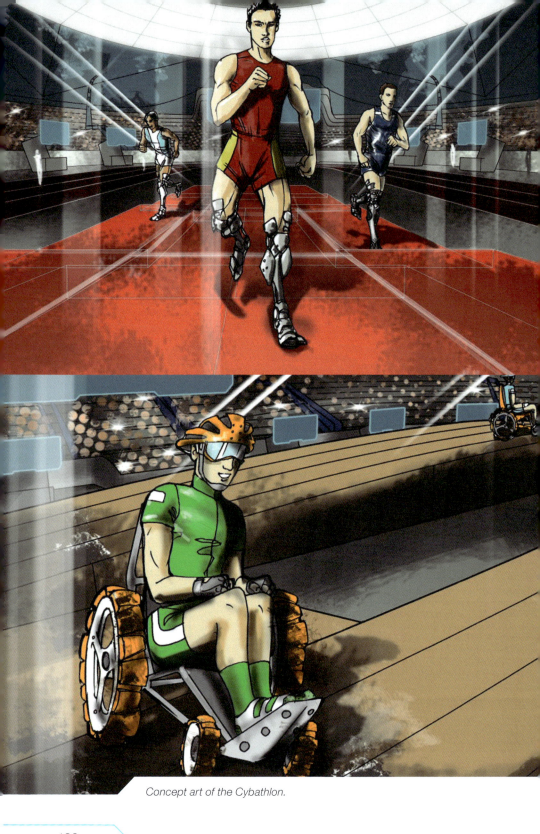
Concept art of the Cybathlon.

The first cyborg ever

One morning in 2004, University of Toronto Professor Steve Mann was awakened by a car that smashed into the corner of his house. He tried to speak with the driver but the driver sped off, striking Professor Mann and running over his right foot. He had been working on wearable devices for 35 years and was wearing his computerized-vision system that gives him a better view of the world. The impact injured his leg and broke the wearable computing system which normally overwrites its memory buffers rather than permanently recording images. But as a result from the vehicular damage, it saved pictures of the license plate and driver who was later identified and arrested.

In the 1970s, Professor Mann explored different ways to design wearable devices when most computers were the size of large rooms and wireless data networks were unheard of.

"The first versions I built sported separate transmitting and receiving antennas, including rabbit ears. Nearly everybody around me thought I was totally loony to wear all that hardware strapped to my head and body. When I was out with it, lots of people crossed the street to avoid me. The future of computing was as much about communications between people wearing computers as it was about performing colossal calculations."

In 1995, he was first to have a passport photo showing him as a cyborg even though he rejected the term "cyborg" as being too vague. He has been working on wearable computing devices since high school in the 1980s when his mission was to create a "digital eye". The Institute of Electrical and Electronics Engineers (IEEE) referred to him as the father of augmented reality and wearable computing. His High Dynamic Range imaging invention is used in nearly every commercially manufactured camera including the iPhone.

In his own Eyetap wearable computer, three simultaneously captured images at different exposures are combined in real-time to produce a view of the world that is as rich in details that can be produced by the human eye. By capturing over a dynamic range of more than a million to one, the user can see details that cannot be seen by the human eye or any currently existing cameras. He and others have been working on an eyeborg system that includes an implantable camera in the prosthetic eye.

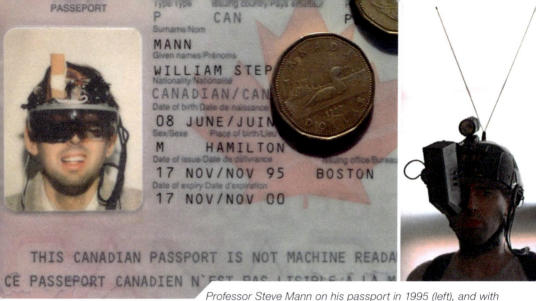

Professor Steve Mann on his passport in 1995 (left), and with one of his prototypes in 1980 (right).

He was also first to make a clear distinction between surveillance (when people are being monitored from a higher authority) and inverse surveillance, for which he coined the word "sousveillance" (when cameras are worn by people). He has written many times that cameras would soon be everywhere, raising positive and negative consequences.

In 2012, Professor Mann wrote about an experience in which he was kicked out of a McDonald's in Paris after employees asked him to remove his headset that could record photos and videos from his point of view. McDonald's issued a statement confirming that he had been ejected, but denied that there was physical contact. Professor Mann, however, released a photo which appears to show an employee grabbing his glasses. He, his wife, and their two children were in line to purchase food when an employee told them that cameras were not allowed. Although Professor Mann presented a doctor's note stating he needs to wear his headgear, employees crumpled up his doctor's note and then allegedly pushed him out the door and onto the street, damaging his gear in the process.

He only asked McDonald's not to prohibit or attack vision research inasmuch as his glasses are designed to eventually help people with vision and memory problems. His case shows with clarity the potential dangers people who wear such technologies will have to face. He also described in one of his papers that wearable device recordings can be similar to human memory, and therefore public establishments should not discriminate against people whose memories are captured by computer devices. He envisions a future in

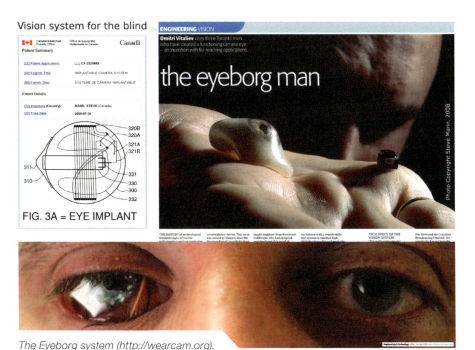

The Eyeborg system (http://wearcam.org).

which people from Alzheimer's patients to healthy adults can use wearable technology as extended memory without being harassed.

Why would society be biased against people who decide to augment their lives with technology in the form of wearable computing or sensors? This is already happening, and there is no reason to think that the number of cyborgs will not increase dramatically in time. Neil Harbisson, for example, recently became one of the first people in the United Kingdom to have a passport photo illustrating his cyborg nature. The color–blind artist wears a head–mounted device called an eyeborg that allows him to see color, and he wants to help other cyborgs like himself gain more rights.

The Most Connected Man

Chris Dancy is usually referred to as the world's most connected man. He has between 300 and 700 systems running and collecting real–time data about his life at any given time. He started five years ago when he noticed his doctor having a hard time keeping up with his health records. Since then, he has lost 45 kg or 100 pounds, and learned to meditate. He told me he is now more aware of how he responds to life and is ready to take steps to adjust to

Trend 20. The Rise of Recreational Cyborgs

his environment. He has also formed better habits thanks to the feedback he is constantly getting from the devices. He gladly shared his views with me.

"We all have beliefs about our lives and our choices. Seeing the data about our lives and choices helps us convince ourselves of relationships we believe we see. With very simple data, for instance, sleep, it's easy to fall into confirmation bias. When you add more data sources such as ambient noise, phase of the moon, air quality, temp, etc it becomes much easier to try to prove your answers WRONG, instead of proving them RIGHT."

Dancy uses a variety of wearable technology from the fitness tracker Fitbit to the Pebble smartwatch, weighs himself on the Aria Wi–Fi scale, and sleeps on a Beddit mattress cover to track his sleep. When I asked him about people's general view about his life, I was not surprised by the experience he's had.

A concept art picture about the most connected man, Chris Dancy.

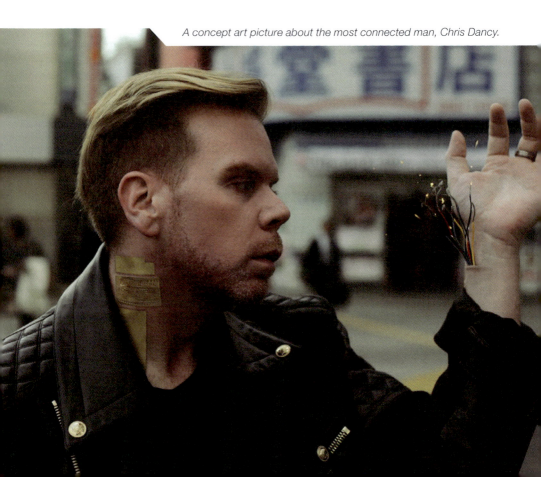

Trend 20. The Rise of Recreational Cyborgs

"Right now it's a bit silly. They either understand and see that my work could profoundly impact humanity, or they think I'm a "gadget nut". Additionally some people on the internet are so very cruel with personal attacks."

He thinks if Apple or Samsung were to add a "health" app, it would be game over for others. Samsung S5 will measure heart rate out of the box. Apple iOS8 will include a health package called "HealthKit,", and the iPhone 5s ships with the m7 chip that is already tracking a person's movements. What is still needed is an awareness of massive tracking and how people could choose to use it for their health and future goals.

In the near future consumers will measure as much data as possible about their health, lifestyle, and other parameters at home rather than in healthcare institutions, and use that data in their health management. Dancy's general view is that within two years most consumers will be in charge of their own health data and many medical decisions, and lower cost insurance

A summary of what parameters and elements Chris Dancy measures and logs on a daily basis.

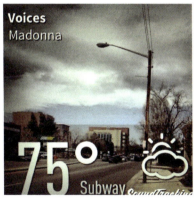

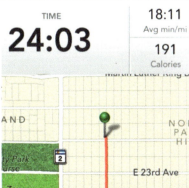

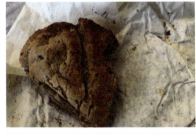

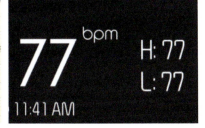

Trend 20. The Rise of Recreational Cyborgs

will be available to those who do this work. As soon as a $100 genetic test is available most people will use their genetic data to manage much of their decision making. He expects to see this common behavior by 2018.

He is looking forward to certain technological developments such as disposable sensors that track motion, skin response, room temperature, humidity, and more, revolutionizing health for people with low income, change the way we experience movies, theme parks, and our very relationship with the people and systems we interact with. Smart clothing that could give us a memory of events from their perspective. Imagine a prom dress that could be so much more magical if it had the ability to collect the experience. But the key is the ultimate health application programming interface as a way for these devices, sensors, services, and applications to talk to one another. Until then, he keeps on measuring a lot of parameters to improve his life.

Augmenting human capabilities

It will soon be possible to be faster, jump higher, think more rationally, be better at drawing, or have perfect eyesight as technological advances make these happen in coming years. What happens when such augmentation becomes commonplace or when we are able to augment even intelligence nobody knows. Moving health disadvantages to normal has been the focus of modern

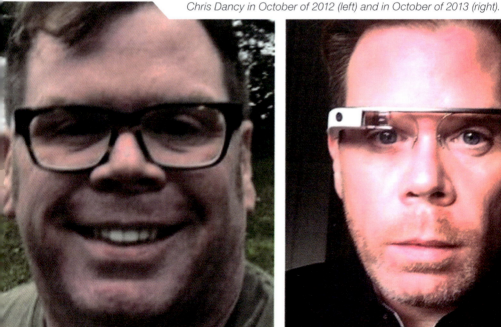

Chris Dancy in October of 2012 (left) and in October of 2013 (right).

medicine. But the upcoming era will be dedicated to actually augmenting these. At what point is there an increased risk of losing what makes us human? When DARPA announced the creation of its Biological Technologies Office, an effort to "explore the increasingly dynamic intersection of biology and the physical sciences", it became clear that we are not far from creating "transhuman soldiers". Quadriplegic volunteers who partially or totally lost the use of all their limbs agreed to undergo brain surgery to have a small array placed on the surface of their brains that picked up neural signals for motor control. They learned to use them to control sophisticated robotic arms. It was a connection between the human brain and the rest of the world.

Does it really matter to what extent we implement technologies in our bodies if it can prevent or cure diseases? Would anyone oppose the extensive use of innovative technologies if it eradicated diseases? Imagine a fully automated "artificial pancreas" that closely mimics the insulin delivery of a working pancreas using technology that continuously monitors glucose levels and adjusts insulin delivery with minimal or no patient interaction. Imagine how the lives of diabetic patients worldwide could improve.

The real challenge is not the advancement of technologies as it is going forward. But from what point should it be considered a threat to humanity instead of a gift? Determining this will be a huge test.

The rise of recreational cyborgs will not only generate new technologies for longevity, but will initiate a dramatic change in the basic structure of society.

Score of availability: 2
Focus of attention: Patients
Websites & other online resources: Cybathlon (http://www.cybathlon.ethz.ch/), Chris Dancy (http://www.chrisdancy.com/), Prof. Steve Mann (http://www.eecg.toronto.edu/~mann)
Companies & start-ups: Glance (http://www.glanceapp.info/)
Books: Machine Man by Max Barry
Movies: I, Robot (2004), RoboCop (2014)

Trend 21. Cryonics and Longevity

Benjamin Franklin wrote in one of his letters in 1773 that he lived "in a century too little advanced, and too near the infancy of science" that he could not be preserved and revived to fulfill his desire to see and observe the state of the United States of America in a hundred years' time. Epic movies such as "2001: A Space Odyssey", "Aliens" or "Prometheus" all featured people preserved at low temperatures to survive a long space flight and later get reanimated. Cryotherapy has been used to treat skin conditions such as warts, moles, and skin tags. Whole body cryotherapy in specially designed chambers has been used as a rehabilitation method for athletes.

In real life, over 270 people have undergone cryopreservation since it was first proposed in 1962. That means they are frozen with the hope that healing and resuscitation may be possible in the future, although many scientists are skeptic about the idea.

Suspended animation was first tried on pigs (which are physiologically very similar to people) in 2002. Researchers replaced the pig's blood with a cold saline solution, cooling the pig's temperature to 10 Celsius (50F). Its injury was treated, and the pig was gradually warmed back up by replacing the saline with blood again. Despite being dead for a few hours, the pig's heart started beating on its own, and it had no apparent physical or cognitive impairment.

Similar saline–cooling procedures were used to reanimate people who have been recently declared dead. This was the background for research performed in Pennsylvania in May, 2014 to test a new method of freezing gunshot victims while doctors tried to save their lives. It is called emergency preservation and resuscitation. All the patient's blood get replaced with cold saline, which rapidly cools the body and stops almost all cellular activity. It remains to be proven whether the method is safe for wide use in emergency departments.

Regulations in this area are tricky as cryopreserving someone before they die can be considered murder. In the US, cryonics can only be legally performed after individuals have been pronounced legally dead.

The Cryonics Institute in Clinton Township, Michigan stores hundreds of cryopreserved people and animals along with DNA and tissue samples. Sub–zero temperatures halt cells from sustaining further damage from external sources. It costs thousands of dollars upon death, plus a one–time membership fee to get cryopreserved. On their website a buyer's guide and a book called "Cold Facts" are available, including details about preparing for the cryopreservation.

Critics have hit cryogenics hard from many perspectives. Bioethicists said that unless it is technically possible to replace all of the water left in a body's cells with glycol, an odorless, colorless, liquid material used in industrial applications like antifreeze formulations; unfreezing a frozen corpse will rupture the cell walls, ensuring that patients become a so-called "corpsesicle". For the moment, cryogenics remains an area of science fiction.

Transhumanist and philosopher Zoltan Istvan went further in arguing that "parents should have the legal right to painlessly put their extreme special needs children into a cryogenic state while they are biologically healthy and have years left on their lives". Such a point of view demonstrates that society has to start discussing these issues now.

How long can we live?

Hendrikje van Andel-Schipper was born in 1890 and died in 2005 at the age of 115. She left her body to science to find out how she remained in relatively good health for so long. Scientists found that about two-thirds of her white blood cells had been made by only two stem cells, meaning that she had "a superior system for repairing or aborting cells with dangerous mutations." To find the biological reasons for longevity, the Archon X Prize, a $10 million challenge, aimed at sequencing the DNA of 100 centenarians rapidly, accurately, and inexpensively. The centenarians donated their DNA to find out whether they have rare genes that may protect them from age-related diseases.

Due to aging, more and more solutions have to be worked out specifically for elderly people. The Stanford Center on Longevity launched a student contest in 2014. Contestant entries included "Automated Home Activity Monitoring", a system for detecting patterns of daily living and generating a call for help when necessary; "Caresolver", a caregiver platform to give caregivers support and facilitate coordination with a larger caregiving team; "Confage", an engaging gaming experience that teaches older users how to better use touch screen devices; or the winner "Eatwell", a tableware set specifically designed for the needs of people with Alzheimer's.

The science of life extension has many names from anti-aging medicine and indefinite life extension to experimental and biomedical

Trend 21. Cryonics and Longevity

gerontology. The point is that some people would like to live longer lives, and research has been generating a vast amount of data in recent years. Approaches might involve anti-aging drugs, vitamin supplements, repairing cells one by one by nanotechnology, cloning replacement parts, genetic modification, or the ultimate step of mind uploading in digital format.

A 2013 research poll in the United States found that 38% of Americans would want life extension treatments while 56% would reject them. What is surprising is that only 4% consider an "ideal lifespan" to be more than 120 years. The longest anyone has been definitively proven to live is 122 years. Jeanne Calment's birth records confirm her birth in 1875. She died in 1997. A person born today can expect to live more than 70 years based on today's actuarial tables. But globally that person will be able prolong his life span to more than 100 years in a few decades. The first human who will live robustly to age 150 is already alive today.

Joel Garreau, author of Radical Evolution: The Promise and Peril of Enhancing Our Minds, Our Bodies—and What It Means to Be Human, sketched four possible scenarios for longevity. In scenario A, the exponential increases in biological, genetic, neurological, information, nano, and implant technologies will have relatively minor impact on current trends in lifespan, health span, costs, hospitals, and health insurance. In scenario B, such advances in genetics, robotics, information, and nanotechnology will succeed in increasing lifespan but largely fail to increase health span. Scenario C features advances in personalized medicine, tissue engineering, organ regeneration, implants, and memory enhancement as well as novel means of peering into the body along with major interventions in heart disease, diabetes, and cancer. Scenario D depicts an immortality that requires technology to advance faster than we age.

Aubrey de Grey is a British theoretician of gerontology and Chief Science Officer of the SENS Research Foundation. He suggested that a cure for aging is within reach in our lifetimes, while the majority of scientists disagree. He put forth his views in Strategies for Engineered Negligible Senescence, a research and advocacy program that aims to tackle issues related to aging. He says that aging is barbaric and should neither be allowed or accepted. To allow people to die is bad, and this is why he works to cure aging. He donated $13 million to the SENS Foundation after his mother died and left him an inheritance of roughly $16 million.

Trend 21. Cryonics and Longevity

In the early 2010s, companies riding the tech wave have turned their attention to prolonging life. In 2013, Google announced the launch of a brand new company called Calico whose mission is to tackle aging and illness as well as to take a big-data approach to speed healthcare discoveries. The CEO is Art Levinson, chairman of Apple and former CEO of the biotech pioneer Genentech. The company has been persuading renowned scientists to join their efforts, although it is not clear what they actually plan to do.

In 2014, a new company was established by J. Craig Venter, leader of the private team that sequenced one of the first two human genomes, along with Peter Diamandis and Robert Hariri. The mission of "Human Longevity, Inc." is to help researchers understand diseases associated with age-related decline. To achieve this, the DNA of subjects from children to centenarians will be decoded and compiled into a database to include details on both genome and microbiome. They hope to sequence the genomes of over 100,000 people per year, with the intent of making "100-years-old the new 60."

Score of availability: 1
Focus of attention: Patients
Websites & other online resources: Cryogenics Society of America (http://www.cryogenicsociety.org),
SENS Research Foundation (http://www.sens.org/)
Companies & start-ups: Calico (https://en.wikipedia.org/wiki/Calico_(company)), Human Longevity Inc. (http://www.humanlongevity.com/)
Books: Countdown to Immortality by FM-2030, Schnall & de Grey
Movies: 2001: A Space Odyssey (1968), Alien (1979), Prometheus (2012)

Trend 22. What Will a Brand New Society Look Like?

The technologies, trends, and changes we've discussed make it evident that society as a whole will undergo serious and sometimes dramatic changes in the coming years. I have had very interesting talks with ethicists, philosophers, and those representing new concepts in medicine. For instance, I discussed the relationship between the human touch and disruptive technologies with Dr. Mairi Levitt, bioethicist at Lancaster University in the United Kingdom. She has firm beliefs about the changing status quo.

"I agree that innovative technology does not necessarily mean the human touch is removed but that is what seems to have happened so far. I think the human touch is now delivered by different lower status people (if at all). Perhaps innovative technology has worked best when the human touch is less relevant e.g. creating new artificial limbs, or better hip replacements.

The human touch– answering bells when patients ring, listening and responding to patient needs, sitting with new mothers to help them breast feed, feeding patients who can't feed themselves etc. – seem to become low status tasks compared with anything more high tech and are carried out when there is time by those on the lowest rung of the job hierarchy. High tech seems to equate with high status."

Dr. Levitt thinks there will be no major problems in technologies gaining acceptance if they can be presented as prolonging lives, improving treatment, and making life easier for caregivers. The real problem will be how the health service can afford them, and how to make the right decisions on priorities so that low tech treatments that help people are not neglected. She argued that the upcoming waves of technological change in medicine could be dangerous if medical students are encouraged to get excited about technology rather than about helping those who are ill. Medical education has to make sure that it trains good medical professionals who can secondarily deal with technology.

Judit Sándor, Director of the Center for Ethics and Law in Biomedicine at CEU, noted that what seems like enhancement for a medical professional may not look like that from the patient's point of view. What is desirable for one person may be entirely inadequate to another.

Trend 22. What Will a Brand New Society Look Like?

"If classifications are merely techno-centric or pathological, important aspects of fundamental rights may be ignored or simply neglected. Therefore I believe that policies should aim, first and foremost, to restore the dignity and liberty of the people affected. This might only involve the goal to increase physical accessibility to the workplace and to sensitize the work environment for someone who is now considered disabled. One should never view, however, (bio)technological enhancement as a tool for substituting the missing social solidarity."

While ethicists help us discuss the issues that extensive use of technologies in medicine might cause, the question is how to predict the next trends, or how to choose those that seem to have the most potential. Ian Pearson is a well-known futures consultant and sci-fi author who made plenty of successful predictions in You Tomorrow. He provided me with amazing suggestions when I started my journey as a medical futurist. He has definite theories about how hard it is to predict the future.

"Picking up on advances on making connections between nerve tissue and electronics, linking that to activity in skin patches monitoring blood properties, and factoring in ongoing miniaturization, you can easily make a short term prediction that we'll have plasters being used routinely to monitor health in hospital wards, a mid-term prediction that we will soon be able to use electronics on thin membranes or even in the skin surface to record and replay sensations, or display our current health state.

In fact, it was already possible to make such a long term prediction in 2001 when we first understood that we could print electronics on paper and that electronic signals could be transmitted via the skin. So depending what level of technology you consider, it is possible to look further into the future."

As advanced technology takes over more of diagnosis and treatment, human caregivers at all levels will migrate more toward the emotional interface role. He envisions that caring will resume its place as the most important role a nurse performs, for example, while doctors will dispense more advice for prevention and self-care. Machines will do most of the analysis. Advancing technology will encourage humans to focus on the human side and let machines do the work. Recognizing that advanced technology actually humanizes people will lead to the better acceptance of technology, and appreciation for the partnership of man and machine.

Technosexuality and beyond

A man named Davecat lives with his wife and mistress, both of whom are Synthetiks––specially designed, life-sized Dolls. Accordingly, Davecat calls himself a technosexual. In this book one of my goals was to demonstrate how society might change due to emerging technologies. While some will not understand how Davecat thinks about his partners, his story represents perfectly the diversity of concepts and theories that will arise in the next couple of years.

One of the reasons he agrees to make media appearances with his wife Sidore and their mistress Elena is to expose the general populace to the concept of Synthetik humans. Incidentally, Synthetik is a catch-all phrase that he started to use to describe both passive artificial companions, such as love dolls, and active ones such as Gynoids and Androids. Because Dolls are becoming increasingly realistic, humanoid robotics is advancing, and society's mindset is broadening, he believes we will see more and more Synthetiks in the next couple of decades. He told me he does what he does to affirm it is not only possible to lead a reasonably fulfilling life with artificial partners, but that he will not be the only one doing so in time.

"Being an iDollator has improved my life, without question. Having Sidore and Elena has enabled me to meet all sorts of interesting people, both within and outside the iDollator community, and make great friendships. As iDollator culture straddles the line between 'lifestyle' and 'hobby', I believe the same can be said once people are able to have their own Gynoid or Android partner.

Technosexuals will be able to get together and show off their artificial partners, and at the same time, learn new and interesting things pertaining to that world, much as people do when they get together for vintage car meets or those who collect Bakelite radios, for example. Synthetiks, and by extension, technology, genuinely do bring individuals together. To those with the right mindset, it dispels loneliness and fosters an amazing sense of community."

People's general view about his life is a three-way split, he says. There are those who think that silicone companions is intriguing and unique; those who already know about Synthetiks through media sources and think having

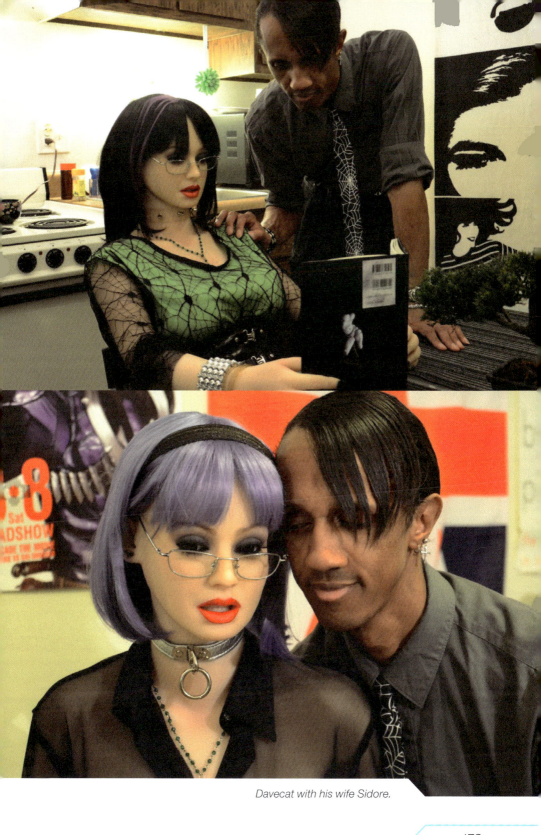

Davecat with his wife Sidore.

Trend 22. What Will a Brand New Society Look Like?

an artificial partner is for losers or perverts; and those who never heard of Synthetiks before encountering him.

"I think one of the reasons that detractors react as they do is due to jealousy. They may have gone through a series of unfulfilling relationships themselves, and seeing someone in love with a Synthetik companion may be upsetting to them. I'm always trying to convince those on the fence about Synthetiks, of course. Both Sidore and I get our fair share of people speaking ill of us, either directly to us or behind our backs on the Internet, but thankfully, we get more responses from supportive individuals, and a handful from those who have seen us on whatever documentary or television segment, saw how contented we are, and decided to save up for a silicone companion of their own."

He agreed that with the right sort of AI programming a person could fall in love with an operating system. Videogames currently exist for handheld systems in Japan that simulate virtual girlfriends, and they are quite popular. Having a humanoid robot that resembles a human would be a sufficient draw for many people, but bestowing that robot with AI would lead to a new society. Anything that can simulate a flesh–and–blood human without any of the flaws or capriciousness of one would definitely be appealing to those who seek that quality. But what about those who are uncomfortable with such humanoids?

Davecat told me he can picture scores of lonely people, whether unlucky in romance, having trouble fitting in society, or elderly people who simply want someone to speak to – better yet a Gynoid or Android with the ability not only to listen but respond – would be a genuine benefit to thousands of individuals.

This story is merely one example of what changes and new concepts society will soon have to face and cope with. In the future we can expect a whole range of new attitudes, roles, and jobs that might sound weird today. A "Healthcare Navigator" might assist patients in accessing information they need in the jungle of healthcare systems. An "End of Life Therapist" might help in planning for the years before a client's death. A "Robot Counsellor" might help wealthy individuals who are looking to purchase robots for their homes determine which model is best suited to a family's needs.

What happens to the millions of prosthetics, breast implants, and pacemakers now in use after someone dies raises not only ecological problems but also represents the range of new problems that must get dealt with. Breast implants and replacement hips are currently not removed at death as there is no clear reason to do so. But cremation is a different issue. Titanium or cobalt implants do not burn up, and any batteries will explode when heated.

To tackle this problem the Dutch company Orthometals collects about 250 tons of such metals every year from crematoriums around Europe. It sells them to automobile and aeronautical industries. A second-hand implant may be the only way that millions of people can afford this life-saving equipment, and so the charity Pace4Life collects functioning pacemakers from funeral parlours for use in India.

With new concepts, technologies, and solutions, what now seem fantastic possibilities will be accompanied by genuine threats to humanity. It is our choice how far we go.

Score of availability: 1
Focus of attention: All of us
Websites & other online resources: The World Future Society (http://www.wfs.org/)
Companies & start-ups: –
Books: Society and Technological Change by Volti; Shaping Technology / Building Society by Bijker & Law
Movies: Metropolis (1926), Blade Runner (1982), 1984 (1984), Bicentennial Man (1999)

Part III: Preparing For the Future of Medicine

Keep yourself up-to-date

No matter how you are related to healthcare, following the main trends of medicine has advantages such as keeping you in the loop of important developments. Try to be up-to-date by using digital methods: subscribing to quality resources and news sites via RSS, or transforming your social media channels into news streams. For example, it took me several months to hide the contacts on Facebook who never post useful articles, and begin to follow pages that covered my favorite topics. Now my Facebook stream is a pure gold mine of relevant information like Twitter and Google+ are. Curation does not only apply for content, but for contacts as well.

Medicalfuturist.com features curated news about the future of medicine every day. It also offers this as a free daily newsletter. Examples of websites covering topics about the future include IO9.com (http://io9.com/tag/futurism), Kurzweil AI (http://www.kurzweilai.net/), and the World Future Society (http://www.WFS.org).

Embrace digital

Whether you like it or not, the world is becoming more and more centered on technologies. It does not necessarily mean that everyone has to agree with all the upcoming changes, or that our lives will all become centered around digital from now on, but accepting the increasing importance of digital is a useful thing to do. Many patients will require a different, more human-based perspective from their caregivers. The needs of these patients, even if the world is fully technological, will have to be addressed. Constantly look for solutions to improve one's practice as a medical professional or one's health as a patient. Time management and certain online solutions might save you a lot of time every week. Embrace digital comfortably and only use techniques that make your life easier and your work more efficient.

Read, listen and watch

No other time of entertainment history has produced as many movies, interviews, and television shows as we have today, or led to the creation of books meant to initiate discussions about the future. Movies such as "Her" (2013) or "Gattaca" (1997), and books such as *Physics of the Future* by Michio Kaku, and Our *Final Invention* by James Barrat speak about ethical issues and considerations we will have to start discussing soon.

Look outside of medicine
Keeping an eye on only medical–related developments will cause you to miss opportunities developing in other industries but which could easily be applied to medicine. What if the next announcement that has a chance to revolutionize a medical specialty comes from nanotechnology, the energy sector, or robotics? Keeping an open eye and informing oneself about concepts not specifically related to medicine could avoid this. IBM's Watson supercomputer or the first nanotubes were not designed with medical applications in mind. But these could still contribute to the advancement of medical technology.

Avoid hype
Hype in medicine has never done anything meaningful. Too much hype can hurt a research area when people realize that the high expectations generated in the early phases have not been met. It took years to get over the hype about smartphone applications. Now, instead of downloading a lot of medical apps, people have gradually learned to choose only the pertinent ones. Evidence backed by massive data is needed for any sensible use of digital solutions in medicine. Checking these studies and papers gives a picture about key research areas. Use Pubmed.com or Google Scholar (scholar.google.com) for this purpose.

Extrapolate from today's trends
Strategically analyze trends and extrapolate the future in a meaningful way. Checking the online resources, databases, books, and movies I have suggested after every trend can help gather more relevant details. Being hungry for new information will be a key feature in the future, and the amount will grow exponentially day by day. Identify which trends seem relevant to your needs. Try to become almost an expert in that. Trend watching is not enough; but knowledge is needed to make your own assessment about technologies, as well as skills that let you choose which trends are the most important ones.

Forget about the ultimate solution
There are movements and philosophies that highlight one concept or approach even though it is highly unlikely that one solution will lead to a prosperous future. A network of interconnected people, devices, and concepts is intended to solve global issues. It is advisable not to trust just one movement or philosophy such as transhumanism or singularitarians. The most plausible solution will be a mix of all the concepts trying to describe the coming

decades. Be skeptical and analytical before accepting major philosophies about the future. In the history of mankind the number of new philosophies has never increased as fast as it is doing no. But it has never been easier to learn more about them.

Don't get scared by the growing importance of technology

Sometimes, the development of various technologies shows a world that is far away from our ideal, but as history has shown it is not common for a particular technology to revolutionize our way of living in a short amount of time. It took over a decade for the Internet to reach its current status; driverless cars have not yet appeared on the roads despite driving millions of miles without incident; and augmented reality devices such as smart glasses or Google Glass have not yet changed the way surgeons teach medical students at thousands of medical schools even though they have been around for years. Such changes will happen eventually, but in medicine and healthcare it takes time to implement change. We need it to properly adjust to new needs.

Don't overestimate technology

When the Human Genome Project was completed people expected that the practice of medicine would be revolutionized within years. It took over a decade to implement the first genomic variants in medical decision making, and it is still a slow and ongoing process. When the iPhone appeared physicians and patients looked forward to using them at home for medical purposes. It took almost a decade for the first evidence–based medical application to get accepted by insurance companies. Technology alone will not provide solutions to the major problems that healthcare institutions face worldwide. It can provide us with tools and opportunities, but nothing more.

Don't give up if you lack IT skills

A lot of medical professionals, particularly older ones, have told me they have given up on keeping track of new technologies because sometimes they even have a hard time turning on a computer. For them, forthcoming solutions will be a huge help given that IT equipment is expected to become simpler in the coming years. By being able to input data into medical records on holographic keyboards and simple user interfaces instead of suffering with antiquated systems will facilitate the job for those who now struggle with technologies.

Fight to keep the human touch
Even though I might sound optimistic given the preface and introduction to this book, the quick rise of technological advances shows the promise of removing the human element in medical practice. This scenario largely depends on how we tackle the challenges we will soon face. Let's find solutions that enable, moreover require, the human touch. While healthcare will become more efficient, medicine will still be centered on people communicating with each other.

Accept mutual relationships
Without a public acceptance of the mutual relationship between using disruptive technologies and maintaining the human touch, the coming waves of changes will only lead to strife. If conservative stakeholders of medicine only want to keep the human touch and spread a feeling of fear against technologies, or if technologists overpromise new devices and techniques, then the outcome will be the least desirable for us all. There must be a balance between these approaches, and I remain confident that by learning about both sides it will become possible to prepare for that balance over time.

Prepare others for the changes
Even in 2014 it is relatively rare to read or watch news segments that depict future technologies and how they could be used in medicine. It is still a big deal when someone mentions longevity, nanotechnology, or surgical robotics in a television program. There is only a small set of online resources covering these issues, their ethical considerations, and potential threats. What would help is discussing such ideas and directions with one another. Spread the word, ask questions, and engage people who are interested in the amazing intersection of technology and the practice of medicine.

Predicting the future of medicine is challenging
Medicine and healthcare represent unique fields that are based on very specific rules, and where new methods and treatments are added to an old basic structure. Nobody can predict the future of medicine in detail, although extrapolating to upcoming years based on current trends is one possible way. As a proof, in the 18th century French painters were asked to paint what the world would be like in the year 2000. Checking the results you will realize these artists had pretty crazy ideas, as well as they hit the nail with some others such

as teleconferencing or fast vehicles. However, they made mistakes assuming that education would be like putting books into a machine that would transfer the knowledge into the minds of students. While it would be beneficial, the approach works better for IBM's Watson than it does for people. As these research trends are constantly evolving, repeated evaluation of the choices we've made is necessary to make sure that the picture we have about the future is still relevant.

Communicate and crowdsource

The end of this book should mean the beginning of many discussions. The whole community talking about the future is interested in your opinions concerning trends that shape the future. Given that a goal of this guide is to initiate public discussions, please feel free to use the #medicalfuture hashtag on Twitter, as well as any blogs and other social media channels to express your thoughts. Influence decision makers if your idea can make a change. Be bold and feel free to crowdsource solutions to complicated problems; use the power of the masses and crowdfund if you have a good idea without the required financial background. There are no limitations for good ideas any more.

Conclusion

"There is nothing like a dream to create the future."
-Victor Hugo

Futurists such as Ray Kurzweil and Ian Pearson usually talk about one of the final inventions of mankind, the digital brain. By the time we understand how the brain works neuron by neuron on small and large scales, we should be able to download our thoughts, our mind, and our memories and live forever in this digital brain. While it won't happen any time soon, I feel that the digital brain has already been invented in my professional life. I call it social media.

Online, I have access to a large repository of expert minds in my fields of interests. I can count on them whenever I need answers or basic information about scientific, medical, or clinical issues. I live within a huge network of people with whom I can communicate constantly. Back when I had a complicated question as a medical student I could ask my professors, fellow students, and maybe make a few phone calls. But often I was alone without an answer. It was a terrible feeling to be left alone when making important decisions. I never wanted to feel that way again. Therefore I spent years creating online networks on my blog, Google+, Facebook, Twitter, and Linkedin to assure that professionally I would never be alone again. Making it possible for every medical professional and patient to say the same line: I'm never alone. This might be the biggest invention in the history of medicine.

Innovation happens faster than ever. Huge companies and start-ups are eager to revolutionize small or large segments of medicine. Patients are becoming e-patients who persuade their doctors to move closer to the digital world. By educating students and medical professionals over time, we can give them the skills to save time in their practices and to be better guides for their patients in this digital jungle. Recent examples have demonstrated the potential and power of technology, and how it can give us better opportunities to connect, learn, and improve as people. What is still missing is a comprehensive, extensive, and public discussion that includes ethicists and representatives of all groups in order to cover the major issues about to shape the future of healthcare and medicine. This book was meant to initiate such debates and, hopefully, it is just the beginning.

Based on the trends and technologies presented in this book, we can assume that no matter how important a role technology will play in our lives,

Conclusion

human touch is and will always be the key in the doctor–patient relationship. Even though the waves of change coming towards us will be huge, and the effects may be devastating, medicine can not only survive but a new system of healthcare and a new way of practicing medicine will be born if all the stakeholders are prepared. Each can make its own assumptions, and acquire whatever skills are needed to adjust to this ever-changing new world. I think we have time, and that it is still possible.

I hope that this book will help people prepare for the amazing yet uncertain future of medicine, as well as a new world of healthcare that optimistically leads to an era when a guide is not needed any more.

Acknowledgements

Ernest Hemingway who won the Nobel Prize in Literature in 1954 said in his acceptance speech that "Writing at its best is a lonely life." I'm very thankful to my wife who made sure this does not apply to me. I'm grateful to my family for bearing with me throughout the long months while I was writing. And I'm pleased to have my friends who kept on sending me amusing e-mails when they knew I was working hard.

Many thanks to Lucien Engelen for writing the foreword for this book; and for providing me with a lot of suggestions and advice over the years.

This book would not be the same without the amazing editorial work of Dr. Richard E. Cytowic; the cover art of Szilvia Kora; and the interior design of Roland Rekeczki.

I cannot be thankful enough to all the experts who agreed to be interviewed for this book, including Jason Berek-Lewis, Dr. Christian Assad-Kottner, Denise Silber, Dave deBronkart, Jared Heyman, Alexander Ryu, Isabel Hoffmann, Mathias Kück, Dr. Rafael Grossmann, Ziv Meltzer, Dr. Arun Mathews, Kimble L. Jenkins, Sarah Doll, Dr. Jur Koksma, Prof. Blake Hannaford, Dr. Catherine Mohr, Prof. Jacob Rosen, Dr. Joel Dudley, Prof. George Church, Dr. Edward Abrahams, Prof. Takao Someya, Dr. Dave Albert, Prof. Robert Langer, Prof. Anthony Atala, Jack Andraka, Michael Molitch-Hou, Mike Renard, Russ Angold, Prof. Robert Hester, Dr. Casey Bennett, Dr. András Paszternák, Conor Russomanno, Ariel Garten, Prof. Robert Riener, Chris Dancy, Prof. Steve Mann, Davecat, Ian Pearson, Dr. Mairi Levitt, Dr. Malia Fullerton, Prof. Judit Sandor, Prof. Ed Boyden and many companies and startups.

I also appreciate the music that helped me write for long hours provided by the Focus@Will team and the songs composed by Cliff Martinez.

Illustration Sources

Page 7: E-Patient Dave deBronkart
Page 16: Wellapets
Page 22: Fotografie Katharina Jäger ©2011
Page 26: TellSpec
Page 28: HapiFork
Page 29: Dr. Rafael Grossmann
Page 33: Eye-On Glasses
Page 38: InTouch Health
Page 45: NerdCore Medical
Page 51: [2014] Intuitive Surgical, Inc
Page 53: Dr. Catherine Mohr
Page 55: Prof. Blake Hannaford, University of Washington, and Prof. Jacob Rosen, University of California, Santa Cruz.
Page 58: H&S-Robots
Page 64: National Human Genome Research Institute
Page 66: Gentle
Page 72: Takao Someya
Page 73: Takayasu Sakurai & Takao Someya
Page 74: Takao Someya
Page 75: MC10
Page 76: MC10
Page 78: Scanadu
Page 81: AliveCor
Page 82: Courtesy of Labonfoil EU Project 224306.
Page 84: Courtesy of Labonfoil EU Project 224306.
Page 85: pApp
Page 88: Prof. Atala, Wake Forest Institute for Regenerative Medicine
Page 89: Prof. Atala, Wake Forest Institute for Regenerative Medicine
Page 90: Prof. Atala, Wake Forest Institute for Regenerative Medicine
Page 91: Prof. Atala, Wake Forest Institute for Regenerative Medicine
Page 96: Jack Andraka
Page 97: Jack Andraka
Page 99: License: Creative Commons Attribution-ShareAlike 3.0 Unported License.
Page 105: Organovo
Page 106: Organovo

Illustration Sources

Page 109: Robohand.
Page 112: 3D Systems
Page 113: 3D Systems
Page 115: Ekso Bionics.
Page 117: Courtesy 3D Systems.
Page 118: Courtesy 3D Systems.
Page 119: Touch Bionics.
Page 125: Timothy.ruban on Wikipedia; license: Creative Commons Attribution–Share Alike 3.0 Unported.
Page 130: User:Clockready on Wikimedia Commons, license: Creative Commons Attribution–ShareAlike 3.0 Unported
Page 132: Casey C. Bennett & Kris Hauser [2013] "Artificial intelligence framework for simulating clinical decision-making: A Markov decision process approach." Artificial Intelligence in Medicine. 57(1): 9–19
Page 144: NXT Health
Page 147: Li Li, Mount Sinai Icahn School of Medicine, and Ayasdi
Page 151: InteraXon
Page 154: OpenBCI
Page 163: D'Arc. Studio Associates Architects
Page 165: Steve Mann, (2013). "Veillance and Reciprocal Transparency: Surveillance versus Sousveillance, AR Glass, Lifelogging, and Wearable Computing" Proceedings of the IEEE ISTAS 2013, Toronto, Ontario, Canada, pp1–12.
Page 166: http://wearcam.org
Page 167: Chris Dancy
Page 168: Chris Dancy
Page 169: Chris Dancy
Page 178: Itagaki Azusa
Page 178: Itagaki Azusa

References

Introduction
Pew Research, 15 Theses About the Digital Future
http://www.pewinternet.org/2014/03/11/15-theses-about-the-digital-future/

Empowered Patients
Yahoo Finance, Genentech and PatientsLikeMe Enter Patient-Centric Research Collaboration - http://finance.yahoo.com/news/genentech-patientslikeme-enter-patient-centric-130000088.html
Crowdmed, https://www.crowdmed.com/how-it-works?category=patient
Crowdsourcing A Mom's Medical Diagnosis: Help is needed!
http://scienceroll.com/2012/07/02/crowdsourcing-a-moms-medical-diagnosis-help-is-needed/http://artisopensource.net/
Research Conducted Using Data Obtained through Online Communities: Ethical Implications of Methodological Limitations, PLoS Med. 2012;9(10):e1001328
Accelerated clinical discovery using self-reported patient data collected online and a patient-matching algorithm, Nature Biotechnology 29, 411-414 (2011) doi:10.1038/nbt.1837
http://www.ted.com/speakers/dave_debronkart

Gamifying Health
Do We Have a Winner? Gamification in Healthcare http://www.healthbizdecoded.com/2013/05/do-we-have-a-winner-gamification-in-healthcare/
Wired, Can Gamification Help Fix One of the Biggest Health Problems You've Never Heard Of? http://insights.wired.com/profiles/blogs/seeking-solutions-to-the-biggest-problem-you-ve-never-heard-of#axzz2wujFwuqb
From gamification to personalized medicine, here's a list of companies pitching at IMPACT http://medcitynews.com/2013/10/want-know-pitching-impact-check-list/
12 Surprising Gamification Stats for 2013 http://www.getmoreengagement.com/gamification/12-surprising-gamification-stats-for-2013
Gamification: Still the Future of Fitness?
http://dailyburn.com/life/tech/gamification-future-of-fitness/
Playing for better health with BioGaming http://blogs.msdn.com/b/healthblog/archive/2014/03/24/playing-for-better-health-with-biogaming.aspx
Wired, Forget the Quantified Self. We Need to Build the Quantified Us http://www.wired.com/2014/04/forget-the-quantified-self-we-need-to-build-the-quantified-us/
Alternate Reality Game Will Turn You Into a Fitness Maniac

References

http://www.fastcodesign.com/3028503/alternate-reality-game-will-turn-you-into-a-fitness-maniac

Wikipedia, Re-Mission, https://en.wikipedia.org/wiki/Re-Mission

PSFK Future Of Health Report (slideshow)

http://www.slideshare.net/PSFK/psfk-future-of-health-report-33393202

Serious Games Transforming Health Through Challenging Conversations

http://seriousgamesmarket.blogspot.fr/2014/04/serious-games-transforming-health.html

Nintendo Wii rehabilitation („Wii-hab") provides benefits in Parkinson's disease. Parkinsonism Relat Disord. 2013 Nov;19(11):1039-42.

The Nintendo Wii as a tool for neurocognitive rehabilitation, training and health promotion, Computers in Human Behavior Volume 31, February 2014, Pages 384-392

Mobile Health News, Eight ways the Microsoft Kinect will change healthcare

http://mobihealthnews.com/25281/eight-ways-the-microsoft-kinect-will-change-healthcare/

Science Daily, Wii-playing surgeons may improve performance on laparoscopic procedures http://www.sciencedaily.com/releases/2013/02/130227183500.htm

How do you solve a problem like medication non-adherence?

http://www.bcmj.org/blog/how-do-you-solve-problem-medication-non-adherence

Why the University of Washington Wants Its Surgeons to Play Videogames

http://allthingsd.com/20130911/why-the-university-of-washington-wants-its-surgeons-to-play-videogames/

Medical News Today, Researchers use Lumosity to identify early cognitive impairment in cirrhosis patients http://www.medicalnewstoday.com/releases/273503.php

Eating in the Future

5 Futuristic Food Trends

http://abcnews.go.com/Health/futuristic-food-trends/story?id=20954898#5

Business Insider, This Test-Tube Burger Could Literally Save The World

http://www.businessinsider.com/cultured-beef-burger-could-save-the-world-2013-8

R.I.'s Food Innovation Nexus seeks to create foods to treat medical conditions

http://www.providencejournal.com/breaking-news/content/20131229-r.i.s-food-innovation-nexus-seeks-to-create-foods-to-treat-medical-conditions.ece

BBC Future, The future of food

http://www.bbc.com/future/story/20140206-the-future-of-food

14 Reasons to Be Hopeful About the Future of Food

http://foodtank.com/news/2013/10/fourteen-reasons-to-be-hopeful-about-the-future-of-food

Engadget, Foodini is a 3D printer for everything from burgers to gnocchi

http://www.engadget.com/2014/03/27/foodini/?ncid=rss_truncated

References

The Guardian, Food trends in 2014: from digital dining to healthy junk food
http://www.theguardian.com/lifeandstyle/2014/jan/06/food-trends-2014-digital-dining-healthy-junk-food
Technology at the dining table, Spence and Piqueras-Fiszman Flavour 2013, 2:16
The Elderly Get the First Taste of 3D Printed Future Food
http://3dprintingindustry.com/2014/04/14/3d-printed-future-food
IEET, Future Technology Could Eliminate the Need to Eat Food
http://ieet.org/index.php/IEET/more/pelletier20130107
The Atlantic, The Man Who Would Make Food Obsolete http://www.theatlantic.com/health/archive/2014/04/the-man-who-would-make-eating-obsolete/361058/
Will Stem Cell Burgers Go Mainstream?
http://www.iflscience.com/plants-and-animals/will-stem-cell-burgers-go-mainstream
IO9.com, Could Soylent really replace all of the food in your diet?
http://io9.com/could-soylent-really-replace-all-of-the-food-in-your-di-510890007

Augmented Reality and Virtual Reality

Science Daily, Special glasses help surgeons ,see' cancer
http://www.sciencedaily.com/releases/2014/02/140210184257.htm
Medgadget, Google Glass App Turns Anyone Into Rapid Diagnostic Test Expert
http://www.medgadget.com/2014/02/google-glass-app-turns-anyone-into-rapid-diagnostic-test-expert.html
10 ways Google Glass could show up in everyday medical care http://www.mlive.com/news/grand-rapids/index.ssf/2014/01/10_ways_google_glass_could_tra.html
Forbes, ,OK Glass, Save A Life.' The Application Of Google Glass In Sudden Cardiac Death http://www.forbes.com/sites/johnnosta/2013/07/06/ok-glass-save-a-life-the-application-of-google-glass-in-sudden-cardiac-arrest/
Medgadget, Google Glass Coming to Rhode Island Emergency Room to Help Diagnose Skin Conditions (VIDEO) http://www.medgadget.com/2014/03/google-glass-coming-to-rhode-island-emergency-room-to-help-diagnose-skin-conditions.html
Researchers develop Google Glass app that delivers instant analysis of point-of-care diagnostic tests http://www.imedicalapps.com/2014/03/researchers-google-glass-app-medical-diagnostic-tests/
Graphene smart contact lenses could give you thermal infrared and UV vision
http://www.extremetech.com/extreme/178593-graphene-smart-contact-lenses-could-give-you-thermal-infrared-and-uv-vision
Continuous Monitoring Contact Lenses - A Moonshot Proposal
http://www.engineering.com/DesignerEdge/DesignerEdgeArticles/ArticleID/6415/Continuous-Monitoring-Contact-Lenses--A-Moonshot-Proposal.aspx

References

The Next Web, How augmented reality is augmenting its own future
http://thenextweb.com/insider/2014/01/31/augmented-reality-augmenting-future/#!Bcn94
Facebook, Google, And Sony Are Getting Ready To Fight A Cyberpunk War
http://www.fastcodesign.com/3027921/facebook-google-and-sony-are-getting-ready-to-fight-a-cyberpunk-war
Daily Mail, Glass without the glasses: Google patents smart contact lens system with a CAMERA built in http://www.dailymail.co.uk/sciencetech/article-2604543/Glass-without-glasses-Google-patents-smart-contact-lens-CAMERA-built-in.html
Medgadget, Personal Neuro Seeks to Combine Google Glass with EEG [INTERVIEW]
http://www.medgadget.com/2014/04/personal-neuro-seeks-to-combine-google-glass-with-eeg-interview.html
Doctor Credits Google Glass For Saving This Patient's Life http://www.huffingtonpost.com/2014/04/10/google-glass-saves-life-steven-horng_n_5120371.html
Breastfeeding Mothers Getting Help From Google Glass?
http://scienceroll.com/2014/02/04/breastfeeding-mothers-getting-help-from-google-glass/
Wearable technology to improve education and patient outcomes in a cardiology fellowship program - a feasibility study, Health and Technology December 2013, Volume 3, Issue 4, pp 267-270

Telemedicine and Remote Care
Smithsonian.com, Telemedicine Predicted in 1925
http://www.smithsonianmag.com/history/telemedicine-predicted-in-1925-124140942/?no-ist
GizMag, iRobot receives FDA approval for physician avatar RP-VITA
http://www.gizmag.com/irobot-intouch-health-rp-vita-medical-fda-approval/25977/
When Life Gives You Lemons, Make Lemonade. When Life Gives You Cancer…
https://medium.com/personal-stories-about-healthcare/when-life-gives-you-lemons-make-lemonade-when-life-gives-you-cancer-b2c9a3d8aa6d
What is the future of telemedicine?
http://blog.econocom.com/en/blog/what-is-the-future-of-telemedicine/
These 4 Companies Could Alter the Future of Telehealth http://www.fool.com/investing/general/2014/02/06/these-4-companies-could-alter-the-future-of-telehe.aspx
Should It Really Take 14 Years to Become a Doctor?
http://www.slate.com/articles/health_and_science/medical_examiner/2014/03/physician_shortage_should_we_shorten_medical_education.html
The Guardian, Telehealth can play an important role in the future of healthcare
http://www.theguardian.com/healthcare-network/2013/nov/12/telehealth-important-role-future-healthcare

References

Deloitte, eVisits: the 21st century housecall http://www2.deloitte.com/content/dam/Deloitte/global/Documents/Technology-Media-Telecommunications/gx-tmt-2014prediction-evisits.pdf

Larry Page Makes the Case for Electronic Medical Records https://www.linkedin.com/today/post/article/20140322154035-19886490-larry-page-on-electronical-medical-records-ted

Robots let doctors ,beam' into remote hospitals http://www.modernhealthcare.com/article/20131117/INFO/311169930

Venure Beat, Practice Fusion owes its success — and its culture — to a motorcycle crash http://venturebeat.com/2013/01/29/practice-fusion-owes-its-success-and-its-culture-to-a-motorcycle-crash/

IEEE, Remote tactile sensing glove-based system http://ieeexplore.ieee.org/xpl/articleDetails.jsp?arnumber=5626824

Physician Shortages to Worsen Without Increases in Residency Training https://www.aamc.org/download/153160/data/physician_shortages_to_worsen_without_increases_in_residency_tr.pdf

Global Challenges Facing Humanity http://www.millennium-project.org/millennium/Global_Challenges/chall-08.html

Re-Thinking the Medical Curriculum

UA College of Medicine Cuts Deal For Synthetic Cadaver http://www.tucsonweekly.com/TheRange/archives/2013/10/31/ua-college-of-medicine-cuts-deal-for-synthetic-cadaver

Medgadget, Virtual Reality Dissection System Helps Study Anatomy, Spare a Cadaver (VIDEO) http://www.medgadget.com/2014/04/virtual-reality-dissection-system-helps-study-anatomy-spare-a-cadaver-video.html

The New York Times, The Virtual Anatomy, Ready for Dissection http://www.nytimes.com/2012/01/08/business/the-human-anatomy-animated-with-3-d-technology.html

Medgadget, Real Time MRI Guidance and Visualization for Brain Surgery Using Clearpoint System: Interview with CEO of MRI Interventions http://www.medgadget.com/2013/11/real-time-mri-guidance-and-visualization-for-brain-surgery-using-clearpoint-system-interview.html

Surgical and Humanoid Robots

Jacob Rosen, Surgical Robotics - Chapter 5, In "Medical Devices" edited by Martin Culjat, Rahul Singh, and Hua Lee, John Wiley & Sons 2013 pp. 63-97.

Jacob Rosen, Blake Hannaford, Richard Satava, Surgical Robotics - Systems Applications and Visions, 1st edition 2011 by Springer, ISBN 978-1-4419-1126-1 http://www.springerlink.com/content/978-1-4419-1125-4#section=841753&page=1

References

Information Week, 10 Medical Robots That Could Change Healthcare
http://www.informationweek.com/mobile/10-medical-robots-that-could-change-healthcare/d/d-id/1107696?page_number=2
Here's a robot that can draw your blood
http://www.dvice.com/2013-7-28/heres-robot-can-draw-your-blood
Medical Robots: Current Systems and Research Directions, Journal of Robotics Volume 2012 (2012), Article ID 401613, 14 pages
Technology Review, Building a Self-Assembling Stomach-Bot
http://www.technologyreview.com/news/410857/building-a-self-assembling-stomach-bot/
Healthcare Innovation and the National Robotics Initiative
http://blog.larta.org/2013/08/28/healthcare-innovation-and-the-national-robotics-initiative/
Wired, Peering under your skin: the future of surgical robotics is virtual
http://www.wired.co.uk/news/archive/2013-06/11/robo-surgeons
Medgadget, Intuitive's New da Vinci Xi Robotic Surgical System Unveiled (VIDEO)
http://www.medgadget.com/2014/04/intuitives-new-da-vinci-xi-robotic-surgical-system-unveiled-video.html
Using Drones to Deliver Medical Supplies in Roadless Areas
http://engineering.curiouscatblog.net/2014/04/10/using-drones-to-deliver-medical-supplies-in-roadless-areas/
Medical News Today, Improving the human-robot connection
http://www.medicalnewstoday.com/releases/275441.php
Daily Mail, Carl the robot bartender serves customers at German bar
http://www.dailymail.co.uk/news/article-2379966/Carl-robot-bartender-pours-drinks-customers-German-bar.html

Genomics and Truly Personalized Medicine

Kurzweil AI, Craig Venter's 'biological teleportation' device
http://www.kurzweilai.net/craig-venters-biological-teleportation-device
Forbes, A DNA Sequencing Breakthrough That Many Expectant Moms Will Want
http://www.forbes.com/sites/stevensalzberg/2014/03/09/a-dna-sequencing-breathrough-that-many-expectant-moms-will-want/
Medgadget, Handheld DNA Analyzer Wraps Up Indiegogo Campaign: Interview with Jonathan O'Halloran, QuantuMDx's Chief Scientific Officer
http://www.medgadget.com/2014/03/handheld-dna-analyzer-wraps-up-indiegogo-campaign-interview-with-jonathan-ohalloran-quantumdxs-chief-scientific-officer.html
Penn State Researchers Create 3D Models from DNA Samples
http://3dprintingindustry.com/2014/03/31/3d-models-dna-penn-state-research

References

The Guardian, Startup offering DNA screening of ‚hypothetical babies' raises fears over designer children http://www.theguardian.com/technology/2014/apr/07/disease-free-digital-baby-designer-children-fears

Personalized Medicine Coalition, The Case for 3rd Edition Personalized Medicine http://www.personalizedmedicinebulletin.com/wp-content/uploads/sites/205/2011/11/Case_for_PM_3rd_edition1.pdf

Body Sensors Inside and Out

A New Wi-Fi-Enabled Tooth Sensor Rats You Out When You Smoke or Overeat http://motherboard.vice.com/blog/a-new-wi-fi-enabled-tooth-sensor-rats-you-out-when-youre-smoking-or-overeating

Smart Embedded Devices: Here They Come http://biomedicalcomputationreview.org/content/smart-embedded-devices-here-they-come

Digestive Diagnostics: Portable, Wearable, Insideable http://ibs.aurametrix.com/2014/02/digestive-diagnostics-portable-wearable.html

IEEE, Putting Electronics in People http://spectrum.ieee.org/tech-talk/biomedical/devices/putting-electronics-in-people

Mashable, Lifelogging: The Most Miserable, Self-Aware 30 Days I've Ever Spent http://mashable.com/2014/03/20/lifelogging-experiment/

Health: Sensing Trouble http://therotarianmagazine.com/health-sensing-trouble/

The Verge, Smart skin patch knows when you need your meds http://www.theverge.com/2014/3/30/5558990/smart-skin-patch-knows-when-you-need-your-meds

Engadget, ‚Wello' iPhone case can track your blood pressure, temperature and more http://www.engadget.com/2014/03/06/wello/

World Future Society, The Future of Biometric Identification and Authentication http://www.wfs.org/blogs/ian-pearson/future-biometric-identification-and-authentication

Medgadget, One Step Closer to the Artificial Pancreas: Interview with Medtronic's Dr. Francine Kaufman https://www.medgadget.com/2014/04/one-step-closer-to-the-artificial-pancreas-interview-with-medtronics-dr-francine-kaufman.html

CNN, FDA approves first bionic eye http://edition.cnn.com/2013/02/19/health/fda-bionic-eye/

The website of Takao Someya http://www.jst.go.jp/erato/someya/en/project

Engadget, Japanese ‚smart clothing' uses nanofibers to monitor your heart-rate (video) http://www.engadget.com/2014/01/30/ntt-docomo-toray-smart-cloth/

Medical News Today, Online game helps doctors improve patients' blood pressure faster http://www.medicalnewstoday.com/releases/276932.php

The Medical Tricorder and Portable Diagnostics

A complete medical check-up on a chip
http://phys.org/news/2014-03-medical-check-up-chip.html
A Revolutionary Portable Lab for Rapid and Low-Cost Diagnosis http://www.mdtmag.com/news/2014/02/revolutionary-portable-lab-rapid-and-low-cost-diagnosis
Techcrunch, Biomeme Wants To Turn Your iOS Device Into A Disease-Detecting Mobile DNA Lab http://techcrunch.com/2013/08/07/biomeme-wants-to-turn-your-ios-device-into-a-disease-detecting-mobile-dna-lab/
The Economist, The dream of the medical tricorder http://www.economist.com/news/technology-quarterly/21567208-medical-technology-hand-held-diagnostic-devices-seen-star-trek-are-inspiring
Portable Lab Enables Fast Diagnosis of Medical and Environmental Conditions http://www.atelier.net/en/trends/articles/portable-lab-enables-fast-diagnosis-medical-and-environmental-conditions_427875
Diagnostics: A Focus on Imaging, Portability, and Regulations http://www.mdtmag.com/articles/2013/06/diagnostics-focus-imaging-portability-and-regulations
Science Daily, Biological testing tool, ScanDrop, tests in fraction of time and cost of industry standard http://www.sciencedaily.com/releases/2014/03/140326142305.htm
BBC News, ‚Star Trek' - The Tricorder
http://news.bbc.co.uk/dna/place-lancashire/plain/A55853012
51 digital health metrics in 2013
http://mobihealthnews.com/27638/51-digital-health-metrics-in-2013/
Wired, A Gold Gadget That Would Let You Stop Heart Attacks With a Smartphone http://www.wired.com/2014/04/clear-3-d-printed-defibrillators-can-shock-heart-without-pads
Techcrunch, Apple Introduces HealthKit For Tracking Health And Fitness Data http://techcrunch.com/2014/06/02/apple-ios-health/
iBGStar® Blood Glucose Meter http://www.bgstar.com/web/ibgstar

Growing Organs in a Dish

Fear of Immortality http://www.slate.com/articles/technology/future_tense/2013/08/aging_polls_and_life_extension_why_don_t_americans_want_to_live_longer.html
TED, Growing new organs
https://www.ted.com/talks/anthony_atala_growing_organs_engineering_tissue
Process Devised to Generate Stem Cells from Drop of Blood
http://sciencebusiness.technewslit.com/?p=17197
Scientific American, Future of Medicine: Advances in Regenerative Medicine Teach Body How to Rebuild Damaged Muscles, Tissues and Organs

References

http://www.scientificamerican.com/article/future-of-medicine-advances-regenerative-medicine-rebuild-damaged-muscles-tissues-organs/
The Future of Regenerative Medicine
http://www.huffingtonpost.com/andre-choulika/post_5200_b_3598945.html
World Future Society, Investing in the Future of Regenerative Medicine
http://www.wfs.org/blogs/james-lee/investing-future-regenerative-medicine
The future of regenerative medicine: Stem cell therapy may be approaching faster than you think http://www.sp-exchange.ca/2014/02/26/the-future-of-regenerative-medicine-stem-cell-therapy-may-be-approaching-faster-than-you-think/
Gel to heal divide between bones and surgical implants
http://www.rsc.org/chemistryworld/2014/04/gel-heal-divide-between-bones-surgical-implants
Science Daily, Living organ regenerated for first time: Thymus rebuilt in mice
http://www.sciencedaily.com/releases/2014/04/140408115610.htm
The Economist, Engage reverse gear
http://www.economist.com/news/science-and-technology/21600356-first-time-mammalian-organ-has-been-persuaded-renew-itself-engage-0
How these London scientists make body parts in a lab
http://dfm.timesherald.com/article/how-these-london-scientists-make-body-parts-in-a-lab/a0240fa12279467740adb7cfe4cef1ac
Gizmodo, British Scientists Say They've Created Artificial Blood for Humans
http://gizmodo.com/british-scientists-say-theyve-created-artificial-blood-1563033374
Technology Review, Implant Lets Patients Regrow Lost Leg Muscle http://www.technologyreview.com/news/526996/implant-lets-patients-regrow-lost-leg-muscle/
Kurzweil AI, Regenerating plastic material grows back after damage
http://www.kurzweilai.net/regenerating-plastic-material-grows-back-after-damage
Scientists Grow Functional Nerve Cells Using Stem Cells http://gadgets.ndtv.com/science/news/scientists-grow-functional-nerve-cells-using-stem-cells-528959
BBC Future, Will we ever... grow synthetic organs in the lab? http://www.bbc.com/future/story/20120223-will-we-ever-create-organs

Do It Yourself Biotechnology

Scientific American, DIY Biotech Labs Undergo Makeovers
http://www.scientificamerican.com/article/diy-biotech-labs-undergo-makeovers/
Wired, This Woman Invented a Way to Run 30 Lab Tests on Only One Drop of Blood
http://www.wired.com/2014/02/elizabeth-holmes-theranos/?cid=18964974
Biotech Alliance to Humanize Pig Lungs for Transplant
http://sciencebusiness.technewslit.com/?p=17636

References

Wired, Biologists Create Cells With 6 DNA Letters, Instead of Just 4
http://www.wired.com/2014/05/synthetic-dna-cells/
This Genius Kid Has Invented A Device That Quickly Detects Water Contaminants
http://www.fastcoexist.com/3030503/this-genius-kid-has-invented-a-device-that-quickly-detects-water-contaminants
This 15-Year-Old Came Up With Software To Hunt Down Cancer-Causing Gene Mutations http://www.fastcoexist.com/3031095/this-15-year-old-came-up-with-software-to-hunt-down-cancer-causing-gene-mutations

The 3D Printing Revolution

Technology Review, Artificial Organs May Finally Get a Blood Supply http://www.technologyreview.com/news/525161/artificial-organs-may-finally-get-a-blood-supply/
Medgadget, 3D Printing Low-Cost Prosthetics Parts in Uganda
http://www.medgadget.com/2014/03/3d-printing-low-cost-prosthetics-parts-in-uganda.html
Baby Heart Patient Saved by 3D Printing
http://3dprintingindustry.com/2014/02/25/baby-heart-3d-printing
Can you 3D print drugs?
http://theweek.com/article/index/246091/can-you-3d-print-drugs#axzz34Qnp52se
Popular Science, How 3-D Printing Body Parts Will Revolutionize Medicine
http://www.popsci.com/science/article/2013-07/how-3-d-printing-body-parts-will-revolutionize-medicine
Technology Review, Heart Implants, 3-D-Printed to Order
http://www.technologyreview.com/news/525221/heart-implants-3-d-printed-to-order/
How a Medical Clinic in the Bolivian Rainforest Might Use 3D Printing
http://3dprintingindustry.com/2014/02/18/medical-clinic-bolivian-rainforest-might-use-3d-printing
The Scientist, Organs on Demand
http://www.the-scientist.com/?articles.view/articleNo/37270/title/Organs-on-Demand/
Anatomically Accurate Aorta Cells 3D Printed at Sabancı University in Turkey
http://3dprintingindustry.com/2014/03/20/3d-printing-aorta-cells-turkey
Hospital Technician Tethers Cables & Saves Hospital Money with 3D Printing
http://3dprintingindustry.com/2014/03/23/hospital-technician-tethers-cables-saves-hospital-money-3d-printing
Mashable, 3D Printing Is a Matter of Life and Death
http://mashable.com/2013/09/05/3d-printing-healthcare/

References

Bone Replacements and Heart Monitors Spur Health Revolution in Open Source 3D Printing (Op-Ed) http://www.livescience.com/43787-bone-replacements-and-heart-monitors-spur-health-revolution-in-open-source-3d-printing.html

Bioprinting Infographic http://www.printerinks.com/bioprinting-infographic.html

22 Year Old Receives Complete 3D Printed Cranium Replacement http://3dprint.com/1795/22-year-old-receives-complete-3d-printed-cranium-replacement/

Medgadget, Scientists on Track to Assemble 3D Printed "Bioficial" Heart http://www.medgadget.com/2014/04/scientists-on-track-to-assemble-3d-printed-bioficial-heart.html

Bone replacements and heart monitors spur health revolution in open source 3D printing http://theconversation.com/bone-replacements-and-heart-monitors-spur-health-revolution-in-open-source-3d-printing-23789

3D Printed Osteoid Medical Cast - Heals Bones 80% Better http://3dprintboard.com/showthread.php?2918-3D-Printed-Osteoid-Medical-Cast-Heals-Bones-80-Better

Kurzweil AI, 3D-printed tumor model allows for more realistic testing of how cancer cells grow and spread http://www.kurzweilai.net/3d-printed-tumor-model-allows-for-more-realistic-testing-of-how-cancer-cells-grow-and-spread

CNN, Artificial eyes, plastic skulls: 3-D printing the human body http://us.cnn.com/2014/04/17/tech/innovation/artificial-eyes-3d-printing-body/index.html

3D Printing Organs, Blood Vessels and All, Takes a Big Step Toward Reality | Singularity Hub http://singularityhub.com/2014/05/05/new-method-to-produce-blood-vessels-in-lab-grown-organs/

Bioprinting a 3D Liver-Like Device to Detoxify the Blood http://www.jacobsschool.ucsd.edu/news/news_releases/release.sfe?id=1512

US FDA Wants An Open Dialogue About 3D Printing Medical Devices http://3dprintingindustry.com/2014/05/20/us-fda-wants-open-dialogue-additive-manufacturing-medical-devices

Life-cycle economic analysis of distributed manufacturing with open-source 3-D printers, Mechatronics Volume 23, Issue 6, September 2013, Pages 713-726

Researchers Have 3D-Printed Blood Vessels http://www.businessinsider.com/researchers-have-3d-printed-blood-vessels-2014-6

Iron Man: Powered exoskeletons and prosthetics

3D-printed exoskeleton helps paralyzed skier walk again http://www.cnet.com/news/3d-printed-exoskeleton-helps-paralyzed-skier-walk-again/

References

Human Exoskeleton, The 'Body Extender,' Is 'Most Complex Wearable Robot' Ever Built http://www.medicaldaily.com/human-exoskeleton-body-extender-most-complex-wearable-robot-ever-built-270576

CBS News, Paralyzed patients hope ReWalk exoskeleton gets approved by FDA http://www.cbsnews.com/news/paralyzed-patients-hope-rewalk-exoskeleton-gets-approved-by-fda/

Wikipedia, Powered exoskeleton https://en.wikipedia.org/wiki/Powered_exoskeleton

The Future Of Touch-Sensitive Prosthetic Limbs: Real-Time Sensory Information http://www.science20.com/news_articles/future_touchsensitive_prosthetic_limbs_realtime_sensory_information-122278

Bionic body no longer science fiction as researchers develop revolutionary new prosthetics, ways to restore sight

http://news.nationalpost.com/2014/01/01/bionic-body-no-longer-science-fiction/

Wired, The Future of Prosthetics Could Be This Brain-Controlled Bionic Leg http://www.wired.com/2013/10/is-this-brain-controlled-bionic-leg-the-future-of-prosthetics/

BBC Future, Prosthetics: Meet the man with 13 legs

http://www.bbc.com/future/story/20140123-the-man-with-13-legs

National Geographic, Revolution in Artificial Limbs Brings Feeling Back to Amputees http://news.nationalgeographic.com/news/2014/02/140222-artificial-limbs-feeling-prosthetics-medicine-science/

Medgadget, Touch Bionics Unveils i-limb ultra revolution Prosthetic Hand With iOS Control App (w/video) http://www.medgadget.com/2013/04/touch-bionics-unveils-i-limb-ultra-revolution-prosthetic-hand-with-ios-control-app.html

Medgadget, Self-Designed Prosthetic Knee for Extreme Sports: Interview w/Mike Schultz, Biodapt Inc. http://www.medgadget.com/2014/03/self-designed-prosthetic-knee-for-extreme-sports-interview-wmike-schultz-biodapt-inc.html

Medgadget, How Next Generation Bionic Devices Will Help Everyone Trek Through Life http://www.medgadget.com/2014/03/how-next-generation-bionic-devices-will-help-everyone-trek-through-life.html

Why The Future Of Prosthetics Is A Question Of Ethics

http://www.psfk.com/2013/10/prosthetics-ethics.html

From Trauma to TED: Boston Marathon Survivor Adrianne Haslet-Davis on Recovery, Care, and Collaboration

http://www.rwjf.org/en/blogs/culture-of-health/2014/04/from_trauma_to_ted.html

BBC News, Rise of the human exoskeletons

http://www.bbc.com/news/technology-26418358

References

Kurzweil AI, Robotic prosthesis turns drummer into a three-armed cyborg
http://www.kurzweilai.net/robotic-prosthesis-turns-drummer-into-a-three-armed-cyborg
Man Compares His $42k Prosthetic Hand to a $50 3D Printed Cyborg Beast http://3dprint.com/2438/50-prosthetic-3d-printed-hand/
Studio photograph of a young girl wearing a pair of artificial legs http://www.ssplprints.com/image/102576/girl-wearing-two-artificial-legs-1890-1910
Engadget, FDA approves a life-like prosthetic arm from the man who invented the Segway http://www.engadget.com/2014/05/09/luke-bionic-arm-approved-by-fda

The End of Human Experimentation

Wyss Institute, Three 'Organs-on-Chips' ready to serve as disease models, drug testbeds http://wyss.harvard.edu/viewpage/484/
Wikipedia, Organ-on-a-chip https://en.wikipedia.org/wiki/Organ-on-a-chip
From 3D cell culture to organs-on-chips, Huh et al, Special Issue - 3D Cell Biology, Trends in Cell Biology, December 2011, Vol. 21, No. 12
Artery chip shows aspirin can't prevent all blood clots http://www.futurity.org/fake-arteries-show-aspirin-cant-prevent-blood-clots/
Kurzweil AI, Simulated human liver achieved in 'benchtop human' project http://www.kurzweilai.net/simulated-human-liver-achieved-in-benchtop-human-project#!prettyPhoto
Kurzweil, AI, Bone marrow-on-a-chip unveiled
http://www.kurzweilai.net/bone-marrow-on-a-chip-unveiled
The Independent, In silico: First steps towards a computer simulation of the human body http://www.independent.co.uk/life-style/health-and-families/health-news/in-silico-first-steps-towards-a-computer-simulation-of-the-human-body-9340781.html
Wired, Virtual Humans will help NHS predict your treatment
http://www.wired.co.uk/news/archive/2014-05/08/virtual-physiological-human
Harvard News, 'Heart disease-on-a-chip'
http://news.harvard.edu/gazette/story/2014/05/heart-disease-on-a-chip/
Microchip-like technology allows single-cell analysis
http://phys.org/news/2014-05-microchip-like-technology-single-cell-analysis.html
HumMod: A Modeling Environment for the Simulation of Integrative Human Physiology, Front Physiol. 2011; 2: 12.

Medical Decisions via Artificial Intelligence

Is it possible to build an artificial superintelligence without fully replicating the human brain? http://www.vitamodularis.org/articles/can_artifical_superintelligence_be_built_without_replicating_the_human_brain.shtml

References

IBM Watson: The inside story of how the Jeopardy-winning supercomputer was born, and what it wants to do next http://www.techrepublic.com/article/ibm-watson-the-inside-story-of-how-the-jeopardy-winning-supercomputer-was-born-and-what-it-wants-to-do-next/#

IBM's Watson Is Learning Its Way To Saving Lives http://www.fastcompany.com/3001739/ibms-watson-learning-its-way-saving-lives By Jon Gertner

Medical News Today, Evaluating the expertise of humans and computer algorithms http://www.medicalnewstoday.com/releases/271345.php

Wired, Why Human-Computer Teams Hold the Most Promise for the Future http://www.wired.com/2014/02/human-computer-teams-hold-promise-future/

Gartner's 2013 Hype Cycle for Emerging Technologies Maps Out Evolving Relationship Between Humans and Machines http://www.gartner.com/newsroom/id/2575515

IBM, I'll take 'Business and Medicine,' Alex http://www.ibm.com/smarterplanet/us/en/innovation_explanations/article/rob_high.html?lnk=ushpcs2

Artificial Intelligence The Future of Medicine? JAMA Otolaryngol Head Neck Surg. 2014;140(3):191

Medical News Today, A supercomputer could change how diseases are treated http://www.medicalnewstoday.com/articles/272975.php

Wired, IBM's Watson is better at diagnosing cancer than human doctors http://www.wired.co.uk/news/archive/2013-02/11/ibm-watson-medical-doctor

Venture Beat, IBM Watson fires its own cancer-fighting 'moonshot' http://venturebeat.com/2013/10/18/ibm-watson-fires-its-own-cancer-fighting-moonshot/

MD Anderson Cancer Center to Use Watson to Help Battle Cancer http://asmarterplanet.com/blog/2013/10/md-anderson-cancer-center-plans-to-use-ibm-watson-to-help-eradicate-cancer.html

Can computers save health care? IU research shows lower costs, better outcomes http://newsinfo.iu.edu/news/page/normal/23795.html

Forbes, IBM's Watson Attempts To Tackle The Genetics Of Brain Cancer http://www.forbes.com/sites/matthewherper/2014/03/19/what-watson-cant-tell-us-about-our-genes-yet/

The New Yorker, Why We Should Think About the Threat of Artificial Intelligence http://www.newyorker.com/online/blogs/elements/2013/10/why-we-should-think-about-the-threat-of-artificial-intelligence.html

Stanford AAAI Talk: Positive Artificial Intelligence http://selfawaresystems.com/2014/03/24/stanford-aaai-talk-positive-artificial-intelligence/

Five Creepiest Advances in Artificial Intelligence http://www.learning-mind.com/five-creepiest-advances-in-artificial-intelligence/

References

IEET, The Singularity Is Further Than It Appears
http://ieet.org/index.php/IEET/more/naam20140327
Wired, Artificial Intelligence Is Now Telling Doctors How to Treat You
 http://www.wired.com/2014/06/ai-healthcare/
Business Isnsider, IBM's Watson Supercomputer May Soon Be The Best Doctor In The World http://www.businessinsider.com/ibms-watson-may-soon-be-the-best-doctor-in-the-world-2014-4#ixzz34WADQJHn
IO9.com, IBM's Watson computer has parts of its memory cleared after developing an acute case of potty mouth http://io9.com/5975173/ibms-watson-computer-has-parts-of-its-memory-cleared-after-developing-an-acute-case-of-potty-mouth
IO9.com, A Chatbot Has ‚Passed' The Turing Test For The First Time
http://io9.com/a-chatbot-has-passed-the-turing-test-for-the-first-ti-1587834715
Medgadget, The First EMR to Integrate with Watson (INTERVIEW)
http://www.medgadget.com/2014/06/the-first-emr-to-integrate-with-watson-interview.html

Nanorobots Living In Our Blood

Top 10 developments in nanodermatology in 2013
http://nanotechportal.blogspot.hu/2014/02/top-10-developments-in-nanodermatology.html
Types of Nanorobots being Developed for Use in Healthcare http://www.dummies.com/how-to/content/types-of-nanorobots-being-developed-for-use-in-hea.html
Kurzweil AI, Robots in the bloodstream: the promise of nanomedicine
http://www.kurzweilai.net/robots-in-the-bloodstream-the-promise-of-nanomedicine
Science Daily, New nanoparticle that only attacks cervical cancer cells
http://www.sciencedaily.com/releases/2014/03/140314212122.htm
The Nanotechnology Revolution
http://www.thenewatlantis.com/publications/the-nanotechnology-revolution
Looking to the Future: Advances in Nanotechnology, an Interview with Travis Earles from Lockheed Martin http://www.azonano.com/article.aspx?ArticleID=3738
Kurzweil AI, Magnetically controlled nanoparticles cause cancer cells to self-destruct http://www.kurzweilai.net/nanoparticles-that-cause-cancer-cells-to-self-destruct
Popular Science, Nano-Robots That Compute With DNA Installed Into Living Cockroach http://www.popsci.com/article/science/nano-robots-compute-dna-installed-living-cockroach
Superhumans Created by Nanotechnology within 30 years
http://www.thatsreallypossible.com/news/852/nanotechnology-superhumans/
Science Daily, Cloaked DNA nanodevices survive pilot mission
http://www.sciencedaily.com/releases/2014/04/140422100021.htm

References

Contribution of Nanomedicine to Horizon 2020 http://www.etp-nanomedicine.eu/public/press-documents/publications/etpn-publications/etpn-white-paper-H2020
Here's a Surprising Look at How Nanotechnology Could Reengineer Our Bodies http://www.policymic.com/articles/89803/here-s-a-surprising-look-at-how-nanotechnology-could-reengineer-our-bodies

Hospitals of the Future
In The Hospital Of The Future, Big Data Is One Of Your Doctors
http://www.fastcoexist.com/3022050/futurist-forum/in-the-hospital-of-the-future-big-data-is-one-of-your-doctors
Forbes, Hospitals May Be Disappearing In The Era Of Health Care Reform
http://www.forbes.com/sites/robertpearl/2013/11/14/hospitals-may-be-disappearing-in-the-era-of-health-care-reform/
Wired, What Would the Ideal Hospital Look Like in 2020?
http://www.wired.com/2013/07/hospital-of-the-future/
Op/Ed: Hospital of the Future Will Be a Health Delivery Network
http://health.usnews.com/health-news/hospital-of-tomorrow/articles/2014/01/14/oped-hospital-of-the-future-will-be-a-health-delivery-network
The Wall Street Journal, The Hospital Room of the Future
http://online.wsj.com/news/articles/SB10001424052702303442004579119922380316310
IFTF, Future of the Hospital: Foresight Engine Game & Public Analysis Report - http://www.iftf.org/our-work/health-self/health-horizons/future-of-the-hospital-game-report/#sthash.XCTUJvBc.dpuf
The Future of Hospitals: Visions of the Healthcare Landscape in 2035
http://www.beckershospitalreview.com/leadership-management/the-future-of-hospitals-visions-of-the-healthcare-landscape-in-2035.html
Forbes, The Hospital Steve Jobs Would Have Built
http://www.forbes.com/sites/carminegallo/2014/03/26/the-hospital-steve-jobs-would-have-built/
The Future of Wearable Computing in Healthcare
http://www.mdtmag.com/blogs/2014/01/future-wearable-computing-healthcare
The Doctor's Office of 2024 — 4 Predictions for the Future
http://profitable-practice.softwareadvice.com/doctors-office-of-2024-0514/
The Charles Bronfman Institute for Personalized Medicine
http://icahn.mssm.edu/research/institutes/institute-for-personalized-medicine/innovation-and-technology/biome-platform

References

Forbes, Global Study Finds Majority Believe Traditional Hospitals Will Be Obsolete In The Near Future http://www.forbes.com/sites/theapothecary/2013/12/09/global-study-finds-majority-believe-traditional-hospitals-will-be-obsolete-in-the-near-future/

Virtual-Digital Brains

OpenBCI wants you to build products with brain waves and 3D printer http://www.3ders.org/articles/20140113-openbci-wants-you-to-build-products-with-brain-waves-and-3d-printer.html

How to Create a Mind, Kurzweil, 2012, Penguin Books, p. 195.

Supercomputer takes 40 mins to calculate a single second of human brain activity http://www.itproportal.com/2014/01/13/supercomputer-takes-40-mins-calculate-single-second-human-brain-activity/

Medgadget, Build Your Own Brain-Computer Interface with OpenBCI (INTERVIEW) http://www.medgadget.com/2014/01/build-your-own-brain-computer-interface-with-openbci-interview.html

IO9.com, What will life be like when digital brains outnumber humans? http://io9.com/what-will-life-be-like-when-digital-brains-outnumber-hu-1529764158

Meet the woman making brainwave control look more like meditation and less like the Matrix http://www.digitaltrends.com/computing/spotlight-on-ariel-garten-the-ceo-behind-interaxons-thought-controlled-brainchild/#!YW9Cm

Kurzweil AI, Real-time MRI-guided gene therapy for brain cancer http://www.kurzweilai.net/southern-californias-first-real-time-mri-guided-gene-therapy-for-brain-cancer

The Wall Street Journal, The Future of Brain Implants http://online.wsj.com/news/articles/SB10001424052702304914904579435592981780528

How the Human/Computer Interface Works (Infographics) http://www.livescience.com/37944-how-the-human-computer-interface-works-infographics.html

4 Hurdles to Making a Digital Human Brain http://www.livescience.com/37068-4-hurdles-digital-human-brain.html

IEET, Mind-to-mind thought talking possible by 2030, scientist says http://ieet.org/index.php/IEET/more/pelletier20140310

IO9.com, Would it be evil to build a functional brain inside a computer? http://io9.com/would-it-be-evil-to-build-a-functional-brain-inside-a-c-598064996/all

Meet the man building an AI that mimics our neocortex - and could kill off neural networks http://www.theregister.co.uk/2014/03/29/hawkins_ai_feature

Telegraph, ,Transhumanists' are planning to upload your mind to a memory stick... http://blogs.telegraph.co.uk/technology/jamiebartlett/100013025/transhumanists-are-planning-to-upload-your-mind-to-a-memory-stick-and-extend-life-indefinitely-are-they-mad-dangerous-or-the-saviours-of-mankind/

References

Extreme Tech, Hackers backdoor the human brain, successfully extract sensitive data
http://www.extremetech.com/extreme/134682-hackers-backdoor-the-human-brain-successfully-extract-sensitive-data

CNET, High-tech headband reads your mind
http://www.cnet.com/news/high-tech-headband-reads-your-mind/#ftag=CADf328eec

10 of the Most Surprising Findings from Psychological Studies
http://expandedconsciousness.com/2014/05/03/10-of-the-most-surprising-findings-from-psychological-studies/#oq3ghvghoVEeWVYH.99

Wired, Inside the Strange New World of DIY Brain Stimulation
http://www.wired.com/2014/05/diy-brain-stimulation/

The Myths, Realities, and Ethics of Neuroenhancement
http://motherboard.vice.com/read/the-myths-realities-and-ethics-of-neuroenhancement

The New York Times, Can the Nervous System Be Hacked?
http://www.nytimes.com/2014/05/25/magazine/can-the-nervous-system-be-hacked.html?_r=0

The Computer That Replicates a Human Brain
http://www.thedailybeast.com/articles/2014/05/01/the-computer-that-replicates-a-human-brain.html

IO9.com, Biotech Breakthrough: Monkeys can feel virtual objects using a brain implant
http://io9.com/5846275/biotech-breakthrough-monkeys-can-feel-virtual-objects-using-a-brain-implant

Wired, Creating a ,morality pill' more a question of ethics than science
http://www.wired.co.uk/news/archive/2014-05/16/molly-crockett-morality-drug

Science, Creating a False Memory in the Hippocampus
http://www.sciencemag.org/content/341/6144/387

Medgadget, Optogenetics Researchers Stop Pain With a Beam of Light
http://www.medgadget.com/2014/02/optogenetics-spots-stops-pain-with-beam-of-light.html

Medgadget, Light-Guiding Hydrogel Brings Optogenetics Closer to Clinical Application
http://www.medgadget.com/2013/11/light-guiding-hydrogel-brings-optogenetics-closer-to-clinical-application.html

Medgadget, Optogenetics Now in Technicolor
http://www.medgadget.com/2014/02/optogenetics-now-in-technicolor.html

Scientific American, Why "Optogenetic" Methods for Manipulating Brains Don't Light Me Up** http://blogs.scientificamerican.com/cross-check/2013/08/20/why-optogenetic-methods-for-manipulating-brains-dont-light-me-up/

The Brain Prize 2013: the optogenetics revolution, Trends in Neurosciences Volume 36, Issue 10, p557-560, October 2013

Interview: Ed Boyden on Optogenetics, Neuroscience, and the Future of Neuroengineering

References

http://blog.addgene.org/mits-ed-boyden-on-optogenetics-neuroscience-and-the-future-of-neuroengineering
Using Light To Control The Brain: How 'Optogenetics' Could Cure Alcohol Addiction http://www.medicaldaily.com/using-light-control-brain-how-optogenetics-could-cure-alcohol-addiction-265899
Wikipedia, Optogenetics https://en.wikipedia.org/wiki/Optogenetics
Method Man http://www.stanford.edu/group/dlab/papers/KD%20Nature%20Profile%202013.pdf
Independent optical excitation of distinct neural populations, Nature Methods 11, 338-346 (2014)
MIT discovers the location of memories: Individual neurons http://www.extremetech.com/extreme/123485-mit-discovers-the-location-of-memories-individual-neurons
IO9.com, A New Technique Could Erase Painful Memories -- Or Bring Them Back http://io9.com/a-new-technique-could-erase-painful-memories-or-brin-1585412300
Independent optical excitation of distinct neural populations, Nature Methods 11, 338-346 (2014)

The Rise of Recreational Cyborgs

Augmented 'Olympics': Championship for Robot-Assisted Parathletes Coming in 2016 http://www.factor-tech.com/health-augmentation/augmented-olympics-championship-for-robot-assisted-parathletes-coming-in-2016/
Quantigraphic camera promises HDR eyesight from Father of AR http://www.slashgear.com/quantigraphic-camera-promises-hdr-eyesight-from-father-of-ar-12246941/
Digital Destiny and Human Possibility in the Age of the Wearable Computer http://eyetap.org/cyborg.htm
IEEE, Steve Mann: My "Augmediated" Life http://spectrum.ieee.org/geek-life/profiles/steve-mann-my-augmediated-life
Exclusive: Cyborg Steve Mann Details Alleged McDonald's Assault http://blog.laptopmag.com/exclusive-cyborg-steve-mann-on-alleged-mcdonalds-assault
IO9.com, The first person in the world to become a government-recognized cyborg http://io9.com/the-first-person-in-the-world-to-become-a-government-re-1474975237
Mashable, Meet the ‚Most Connected Man' in the World http://mashable.com/2014/03/13/most-connected-man-in-world-chris-dancy
Superhero Vision Coming in Graphene Contact Lenses? http://news.discovery.com/tech/biotechnology/superhero-vision-coming-in-graphene-contact-lenses-140319.htm
DARPA's new biotechnology lab will focus on cyborg tech http://www.dvice.com/2014-4-1/darpas-new-biotechnology-lab-will-focus-cyborg-tech

References

Medgadget, One Step Closer to the Artificial Pancreas: Interview with Medtronic's Dr. Francine Kaufman http://www.medgadget.com/2014/04/one-step-closer-to-the-artificial-pancreas-interview-with-medtronics-dr-francine-kaufman.html

IO9.com, DARPA's New Biotech Division Wants To Create A Transhuman Future http://io9.com/darpas-new-biotech-division-wants-to-create-a-transhum-1556857603/+georgedvorsky

Michigan Man Among 1st To Get ‚Bionic Eye'
http://www.manufacturing.net/news/2014/04/michigan-man-among-1st-to-get-bionic-eye

Graphene Contact Lenses Let You See in the Dark
http://nanotechportal.blogspot.ca/2014/05/graphene-contact-lenses-let-you-see-in.html?m=1

Steve Mann (2013). „Vision 2.0, My Augmediated Life", IEEE Spectrum, Volume 50, Issue 3, Digital Object Identifier: 10.1109/MSPEC.2013.6471058, pp42-47. See also „My Augmediated Life: What I've learned from 35 years of wearing computerized eyewear", http://spectrum.ieee.org/geek-life/profiles/steve-mann-my-augmediated-life

How McDonaldized surveillance creates a monopoly on sight that chills AR and smartphone development Steve Mann, 2012, 1010 (October 10) http://eyetap.blogspot.ca/2012/10/mcveillance-mcdonaldized-surveillance.html

Cryonics and Longevity

Wikipedia, Cryonics https://en.wikipedia.org/wiki/Cryonics

Cryonics Could Help Improve Some Lives in the Future http://www.psychologytoday.com/blog/the-transhumanist-philosopher/201405/cryonics-could-help-improve-some-lives-in-the-future

Wikipedia, Cryotherapy https://en.wikipedia.org/wiki/Cryotherapy

The Verge, Watch these men take care of the frozen dead http://www.theverge.com/2014/4/10/5599668/we-will-live-again-tribeca-film-festival-selection-about-cryopreservation

Cryonics and the search for 'something more' beyond death http://news.nationalpost.com/2013/10/25/cryonics-and-the-search-for-something-more-beyond-death/

Humans will be kept between life and death in the first suspended animation trials http://www.extremetech.com/extreme/179296-humans-will-be-kept-between-life-and-death-in-the-first-suspended-animation-trials

BBC Future, Human hibernation: Secrets behind the big sleep http://www.bbc.com/future/story/20140505-secrets-behind-the-big-sleep

Wikipedia, Life extension https://en.wikipedia.org/wiki/Life_extension

Drooling on Your Shoes or Living Long and Prospering? http://www.slate.com/articles/technology/future_tense/2013/09/four_scenarios_for_our_future_lifespans.html

References

With Calico, Google looks to make your lifespan its business http://www.extremetech.com/extreme/166858-with-calico-google-looks-to-make-your-lifespan-its-business
Immortality, biotechnology, and the woefully unprepared criminal justice system http://www.extremetech.com/extreme/178859-immortality-biotechnology-and-the-woefully-unprepared-criminal-justice-system
CNN, How Google's Calico aims to fight aging and ,solve death'
http://edition.cnn.com/2013/10/03/tech/innovation/google-calico-aging-death/
Boosting Longevity with Massive Genome Sequencing and Cyborg Technology http://www.prophecynewswatch.com/2014/March18/184.html#9172ADeFRplrQoZV.99
Medgadget, Winners of Stanford Center on Longevity's Design Challenge Announced http://www.medgadget.com/2014/04/winners-of-stanford-center-on-longevitys-design-challenge-announced.html
Popular Science, Hints To Longevity Found In Blood Of 115-Year-Old Woman http://www.popsci.com/article/science/hints-longevity-found-blood-115-year-old-woman
XPRIZE 100 Over 100 Candidates http://genomics.xprize.org/100-over-100
Strategies for Engineered Negligible Senescence https://www.fightaging.org/archives/2004/11/strategies-for-engineered-negligible-senescence.php
Interview with Aubrey de Grey, PhD
http://www.lef.org/magazine/mag2013/jul2013_Interview-with-Aubrey-de-Grey-PhD_01.htm

What Will a Brand New Society Look Like?

The Atlantic, Married to a Doll: Why One Man Advocates Synthetic Love
http://www.theatlantic.com/health/archive/2013/09/married-to-a-doll-why-one-man-advocates-synthetic-love/279361/
As Technology Marches Forward, Who Gets Left Behind?
http://footnote1.com/as-technology-marches-forward-who-gets-left-behind/
BBC Future, What happens to prosthetics and implants after you die?
http://www.bbc.com/future/story/20140311-body-parts-that-live-after-death
Mashable, 10 Crazy Jobs That Will Exist in the Future
http://mashable.com/2014/04/28/jobs-of-the-future

Notes

Notes

Printed in Poland
by Amazon Fulfillment
Poland Sp. z o.o., Wrocław

The Eden Circular

Kirkby Stephen ar

Length:	Ascent	
21km (13 miles)	330m (1,083 ft)	6½ hours

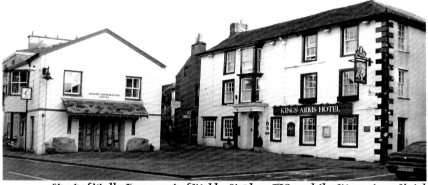

Start of Walk: Forecourt of Kirkby Stephen TIC and the Kings Arms Hotel

Starting from:
Kirkby Stephen Centre on the forecourt of the Tourist Information Centre (TIC) and the Kings Arms Hotel alongside the A685 road. *GR775 087*

Refreshments and accommodation:
Eating, drinking and overnight accommodation are available in Kirkby Stephen. Public House and overnight accommodation are also available close to the route in Ravenstonedale.

Getting there:
Kirkby Stephen is located on the A685 road approximately 19 km (12 miles) from the M6 Motorway at Junction 38 (Tebay) and 6.5 km (4 miles) from the A66 Trunk Road at Brough. Car parking is available in the town close to the start point of the walk, but during the summer months the all day facilities are along roads parallel with the town centre. Regular bus services from Penrith, Kendal and Kirkby Stephen Station serve the town.

Getting started:
The walk starts from the forecourt of the Tourist Information Centre, Market Street, close to the Market Square. With your back to the TIC entrance proceed along Market Street for a few yards then cross over to the front of the Black Bull Hotel. Pass through the archway on the right side of the hotel and shortly reach Faraday Road, the back road parallel to Market Street, and turn left along the pavement of the back road.

Map:
Ordnance Survey 1:25000 scale Explorer Map –
OL19: Howgill Fells & Upper Eden Valley

Eden Wheel:
Kirkby Stephen, Intake Bottom, Moor End, Ash Fell, Garshill, Smardale Gill, Smardale Fell, and Greenriggs Circular Walk

Starting from Kirkby Stephen Centre on the forecourt of the Tourist Information Centre and the Kings Arms Hotel alongside the A685 road. *GR775 087*

1. Kirkby Stephen to Halfpenny House

a) With your back to the Tourist Information Centre entrance, proceed along the main street for a few yards and cross over to the front of the Black Bull Hotel. Pass through the archway on the right side of the hotel and shortly reach the back road, Faraday Road. **(See Kirkby Stephen Centre Route Inset)**

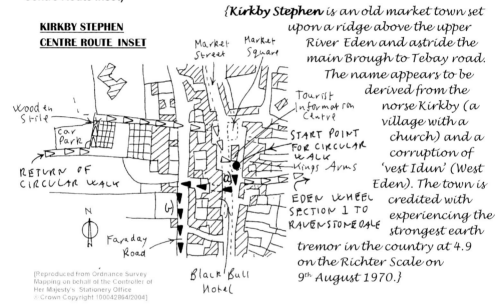

{Kirkby Stephen is an old market town set upon a ridge above the upper River Eden and astride the main Brough to Tebay road. The name appears to be derived from the norse Kirkby (a village with a church) and a corruption of 'vest Idun' (West Eden). The town is credited with experiencing the strongest earth tremor in the country at 4.9 on the Richter Scale on 9th August 1970.}

b) Turn left along the pavement of Faraday Road and follow this across junctions with Fletcher Hill Park, Westgarth Road and Westgarth Avenue. Continue ahead as the road loses its pavement and becomes Croglam Lane.

c) Pass a public footpath sign identifying Smardale Fell and the Coast to Coast walk, then proceed ahead as the metalling ceases along a rough track. The route rises gently and passes a small residential close and the head of Rowgate on the left.

d) Continue along the track, which has once again become metalled, for a further short distance to reach a stone step stile on the left on a path signed to Intake Bottom.

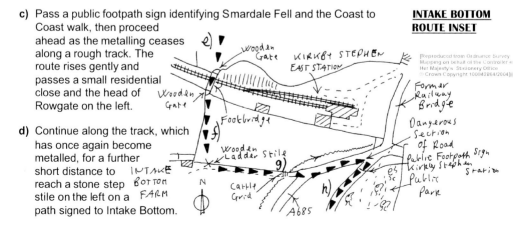

e) Climb over the stile, then proceed in broadly the same direction as before, on a path that contours around the base of a hill, Croglam Castle Hill. Pass through a gated stone gap stile and continue contouring in the next field to reach a wooden gate at the entrance to a bridge over a railway. **(See Intake Bottom Route Inset)**

{*Croglam Castle* is the oval enclosure of an ancient village settlement. It is 0.6 hectare (1½ acres) in area and contains a ditch and external bank.}

f) Pass through the gate, cross the railway bridge (over Kirkby Stephen East station yard), then through a second gate to continue along the right side of a field. At the far side reach a somewhat complex ladder stile arrangement over a stone wall at Intake Bottom Farm.

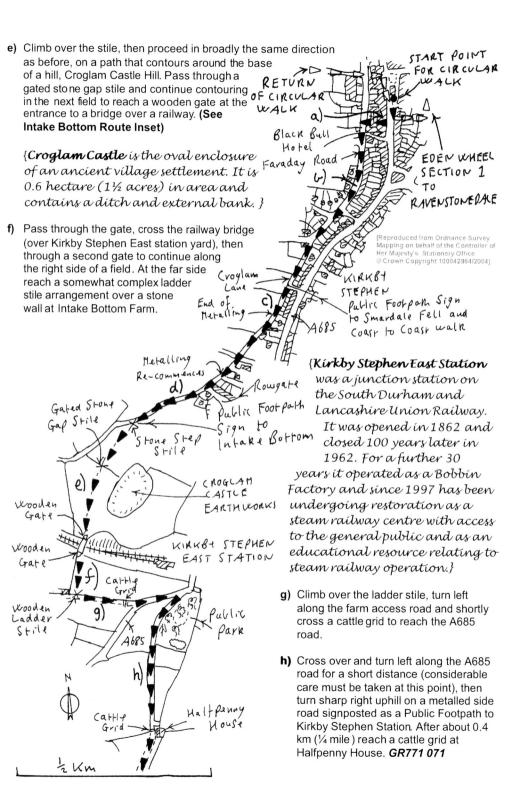

{*Kirkby Stephen East Station* was a junction station on the South Durham and Lancashire Union Railway. It was opened in 1862 and closed 100 years later in 1962. For a further 30 years it operated as a Bobbin Factory and since 1997 has been undergoing restoration as a steam railway centre with access to the general public and as an educational resource relating to steam railway operation.}

g) Climb over the ladder stile, turn left along the farm access road and shortly cross a cattle grid to reach the A685 road.

h) Cross over and turn left along the A685 road for a short distance (considerable care must be taken at this point), then turn sharp right uphill on a metalled side road signposted as a Public Footpath to Kirkby Stephen Station. After about 0.4 km (¼ mile) reach a cattle grid at Halfpenny House. **GR771 071**

2. Halfpenny House to Windy Hill, Ash Fell Edge

a) Continue along a concrete road which is signposted as a Public Bridleway to Birkett Common and Bull Gill. After a further 0.4 km (¼ mile) and a second cattle grid turn off to the right through a metal gate with adjoining wooden stile onto a rough track with a small woodland on the left side.

b) Pass through a second metal gate then after a short rise of the track veer off left as directed by a yellow footpath direction indicator. Cross over a depression, somewhat on the diagonal, to reach a wooden stile in the fence on the far side.

c) After climbing over the stile keep the line of the fence on the right, then when the fence turns to the left and finishes abruptly continue uphill on its line, with odd remains of fencing discernible on the right. Eventually pass over a hill shoulder and reach a further wooden stile in a right hand field corner close to the Settle-Carlisle railway. **(See Moor End Railway Route Inset)**

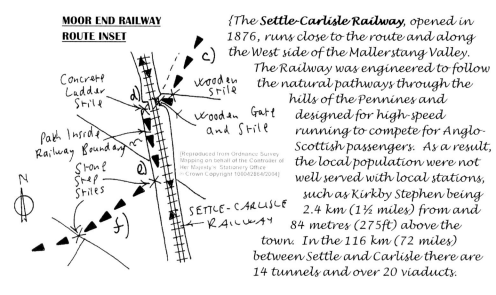

*{The **Settle-Carlisle Railway**, opened in 1876, runs close to the route and along the West side of the Mallerstang Valley. The Railway was engineered to follow the natural pathways through the hills of the Pennines and designed for high-speed running to compete for Anglo-Scottish passengers. As a result, the local population were not well served with local stations, such as Kirkby Stephen being 2.4 km (1½ miles) from and 84 metres (275ft) above the town. In the 116 km (72 miles) between Settle and Carlisle there are 14 tunnels and over 20 viaducts.*

Construction took 7 years and involved 6,000 men and was the last main line railway in England constructed almost entirely by hand. Many died while building the line through outbreaks of smallpox, as well as being killed during construction.}

d) Climb over the stile (and possibly additional wire fencing) then turn right and over a second stile. Pass under the railway then immediately climb over a concrete ladder stile on the left into railway enclosed land at the foot of the railway embankment.

e) Follow along the foot of the railway embankment with a stone wall on the immediate right. After a short distance climb over a stone step stile in this wall.

f) After climbing over the stile proceed ahead away from the railway towards Moor End farmstead. Cross a field to a further stone step stile then another field to a metal gate just to the right of the farmstead. **GR763 057**

g) Pass through the gate and turn right along a metalled road for a short distance, then off left on a rough track to a metal gate.

h) Pass through the gate, then follow the track onto open moorland, with a stone wall on the left containing two field barns within sections close to the track. After passing the second of these barns, veer off to the right to gradually approach, then follow a wall line on the right.

i) Upon picking up the right side wall line follow this across the moorland for about 0.8 km (½ mile) to reach the metalled road that links Mallerstang with the A683 road.
GR763 038

j) Turn right along this road, cross a cattle grid and continue uphill for about 0.4 km (¼ mile) to reach the A683 road. Turn left along the side of this road and cross a further cattle grid onto another stretch of open moorland.

k) Immediately after crossing the cattle grid turn right onto the moorland and with a wall on the right side proceed uphill along Ash Fell Edge to the summit of Windy Hill (385m/1263ft).

{*There has been considerable quarrying along **Ash Fell Edge**. Red sandstone was incorporated into bridge structures on the Settle-Carlisle Railway and limestone was used for lime making and wall building.*}

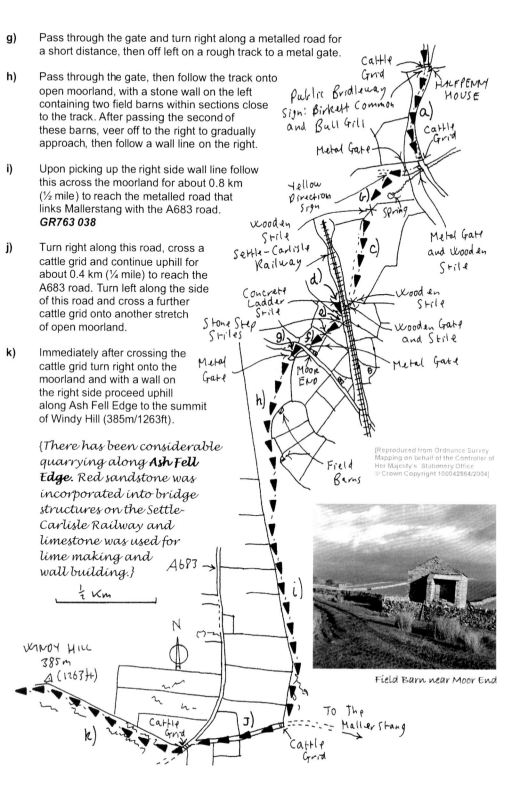

Field Barn near Moor End

3. Windy Hill, Ash Fell Edge to Smardale Bridge

a) From the top of Windy Hill (with the triangulation pillar on the far side of the wall), proceed ahead, turning with the wall, to reach the prominent viewpoint and standard known as Jack's Cairn. **GR744 041** Continue along the Edge, with the wall on the immediate right to shortly reach a wide stone seat, the Paul & Janet Thomas seat, formed within the exposed limestone

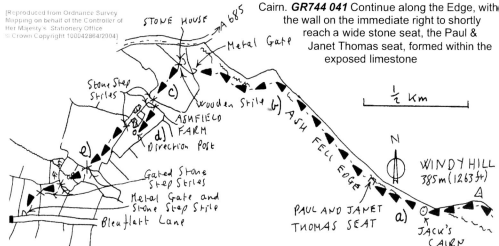

{Jack's Cairn was built by Jack Bradberry, a resident of Ravenstonedale who became their oldest inhabitant and died in 2000. The Paul & Janet Thomas Seat is a stone seat constructed by these regular holidaymakers to the area which is placed to catch the dramatic views west down the Lune Valley and sunset over the Lakeland peaks.}

b) After leaving the seat continue further along the Edge, but descending a little with the wall still on the right to a low point after about 0.4 km (¼ mile) where it turns to the left. At this point veer left and proceed along a path that contours the hill below the wall. Once round the corner of this hill drop down towards the left to reach a metal gate in the wall that is now rising uphill to the left.

c) Pass through this gate to reach, in a short distance on the right, a hollowed out storage byre in the rock, known as 'The Stone House'. Turn left at the byre, climb over a wooden stile and proceed downhill across a field to reach a stone step stile at the far lower side close to a farm.

d) Climb over this stile to a wide sunken track then cross diagonally left to climb over a further such stile on the other side into a field. Follow this path (a permitted path) downhill as it skirts to the left of Ashfield Farm then turn right uphill at a direction post, just past the farm, to reach a stone step stile.

e) Climb over the stile and turn left downhill along the left edge of a field veering slightly to the right to a gated stone step stile in the valley bottom. Climb over this stile and cross the valley (on the right diagonal) through a wall gap by springs then rise up again to the left of woodland. Climb over two gated stone step stiles when crossing two fields, veering left in the second to reach a metal gate and stone step stile at Bleaflatt Lane

f) Turn right along Bleaflatt Lane and after about 0.4 km (¼ mile) reach a 'T' junction with Low Lane. Turn right for a short distance past barn premises and when this Lane veers downhill to the left continue straight ahead onto a rough grassy track signposted as Hobs Lane to Garshill.

g) Proceed along the Lane, with the village of Ravenstonedale visible to the left, to shortly reach Garshill hamlet on the old Kirkby Stephen to Tebay road. Turn left onto this road and almost immediately off to the right over a stone step stile on a footpath signed to Smardale.

h) Proceed ahead on this footpath over a field and cross a footbridge over Keld Sike. Rise up the field to climb over a further stone step stile upon reaching the cutting of the A685 road as it by passes Ravenstonedale.

i) Cross over the A685 road and a further stone step stile at the top of the cutting, again on a footpath signposted to Smardale. Proceed ahead up a grassy track to a further such stile beside a metal gate.

j) Climb over the stile, pass some farm buildings then continue ahead on the right side of pastureland. After a short distance veer to the left, away from the wall and cross over to a wooden gate in the far left corner of the pasture alongside woodland on the right.

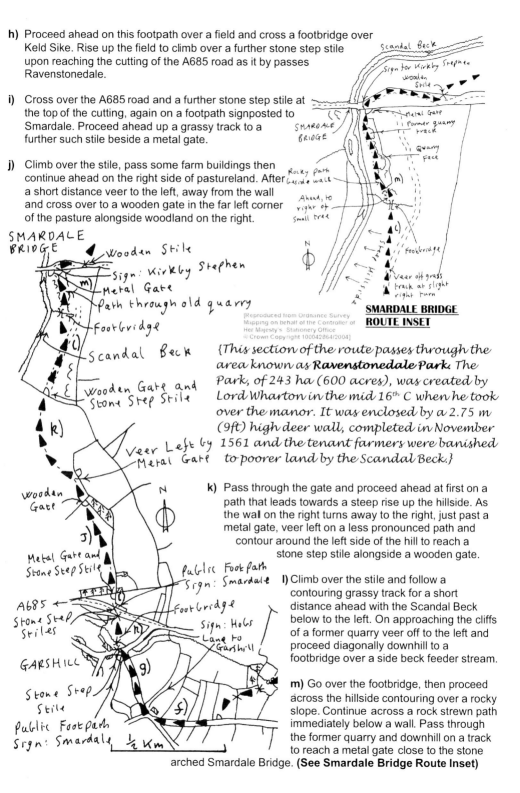

SMARDALE BRIDGE ROUTE INSET

{This section of the route passes through the area known as **Ravenstonedale Park**. The Park, of 243 ha (600 acres), was created by Lord Wharton in the mid 16th C when he took over the manor. It was enclosed by a 2.75 m (9ft) high deer wall, completed in November 1561 and the tenant farmers were banished to poorer land by the Scandal Beck.}

k) Pass through the gate and proceed ahead at first on a path that leads towards a steep rise up the hillside. As the wall on the right turns away to the right, just past a metal gate, veer left on a less pronounced path and contour around the left side of the hill to reach a stone step stile alongside a wooden gate.

l) Climb over the stile and follow a contouring grassy track for a short distance ahead with the Scandal Beck below to the left. On approaching the cliffs of a former quarry veer off to the left and proceed diagonally downhill to a footbridge over a side beck feeder stream.

m) Go over the footbridge, then proceed across the hillside contouring over a rocky slope. Continue across a rock strewn path immediately below a wall. Pass through the former quarry and downhill on a track to reach a metal gate close to the stone arched Smardale Bridge. **(See Smardale Bridge Route Inset)**

4. Smardale Bridge to Waitby Common

a) Turn right after passing through the gate on a rough track, signposted for Kirkby Stephen, leading away from the bridge. Follow this track for a short distance to a wooden stile in the left wall that leads to a nature walk.

b) Pass through the gate, then follow a grassy waymarked path along the edge of Smardale Gill. Pass alongside old quarry workings then rise up gradually on the right side of the Gill towards the restored 14 arched Smardale Gill Viaduct.

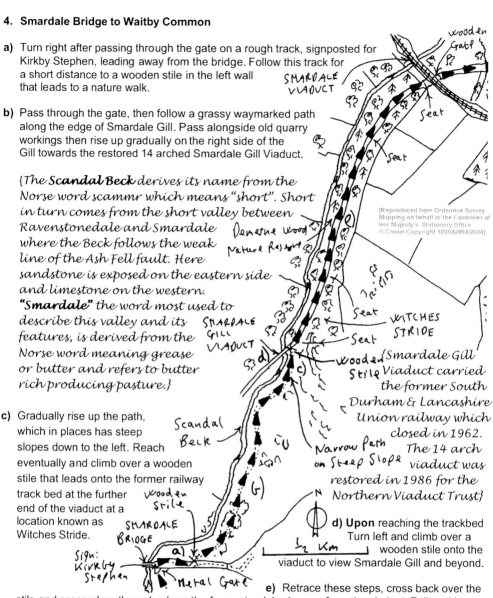

{The **Scandal Beck** derives its name from the Norse word *scammr* which means "short". Short in turn comes from the short valley between Ravenstonedale and Smardale where the Beck follows the weak line of the Ash Fell fault. Here sandstone is exposed on the eastern side and limestone on the western. "**Smardale**" the word most used to describe this valley and its features, is derived from the Norse word meaning grease or butter and refers to butter rich producing pasture.}

c) Gradually rise up the path, which in places has steep slopes down to the left. Reach eventually and climb over a wooden stile that leads onto the former railway track bed at the further end of the viaduct at a location known as Witches Stride.

{Smardale Gill Viaduct carried the former South Durham & Lancashire Union railway which closed in 1962. The 14 arch viaduct was restored in 1986 for the Northern Viaduct Trust}

d) Upon reaching the trackbed Turn left and climb over a wooden stile onto the viaduct to view Smardale Gill and beyond.

e) Retrace these steps, cross back over the stile and proceed northwards along the former track bed, away from the viaduct. Follow this as it passes through the Smardale Gill National Nature Reserve to reach a wooden gate beneath an arch of the Settle-Carlisle Railway's Smardale Viaduct.

{The **Nature Reserve** extends to 42.7 ha (105 acres) and includes grassland, woodland, riverside areas and rock outcrops. It is particularly important in relation to limestone habitats. The 12 arch **Smardale Viaduct** is the highest on the Settle-Carlisle Railway at 39.6m (130ft) in height. The viaduct is built of limestone and because of the clay bed of the Scandal at this point some of the bases reach to 13.7m (45ft) below the ground level of the Beck.}

f) Pass through the gate and continue along the former track bed as it turns and leaves Smardale Gill along a wooded embankment. After about 0.4 km (¼ mile) reach the end of the Nature reserve through a small wooden gate at Smardale. **(See Smardale Route Inset)**

g) Pass through the gate, then turn left up a track to a 'T' junction with a metalled road. Turn right along this road for a short distance and at a further 'T' junction turn right over a 'filled in' railway bridge alongside the former Smardale Halt.

h) After crossing the 'bridge' turn right at a further road junction on a metalled cul-de-sac road signed as a Public Bridleway to the Smardale Fells. Follow this road as it passes Smardale Hall, then beneath the Settle-Carlisle Railway to reach a wooden gate at the road end by dwellings.

{Smardale Hall is of 16th Century origin and has four round towers with conical roofs like a Scottish castle. It now forms the centre of a farmstead.}

i) Pass through this gate onto a rough track signed as a Public Bridleway to Brownber and the A685. Follow this track steeply uphill, turning sharply to the right then passing alongside a plantation on the right side to reach a wooden gate on the hillside slope. **GR738 075**

j) Pass through the gate and continue uphill across pastureland to a second metal gate onto open fell. Immediately after passing through this gate turn sharply left and proceed uphill with a wall on the left, to eventually reach the high point on the shoulder of Smardale Fell.

k) After reaching this high point turn with the wall and continue ahead with a prominent fell route joining from the right. Proceed downhill, over Waitby Common, with the wall still on the left, to reach a metal gate and wooden ladder stile at a corner on the metalled Waitby to A685 road at the edge of Waitby Common.

l) Turn right along the road and after a short distance turn left at a 'T' junction on a road signed to Waitby. After a similar short distance turn off right over a stone step stile signed as a Public Footpath for Kirkby Stephen and the Coast to Coast Walk.

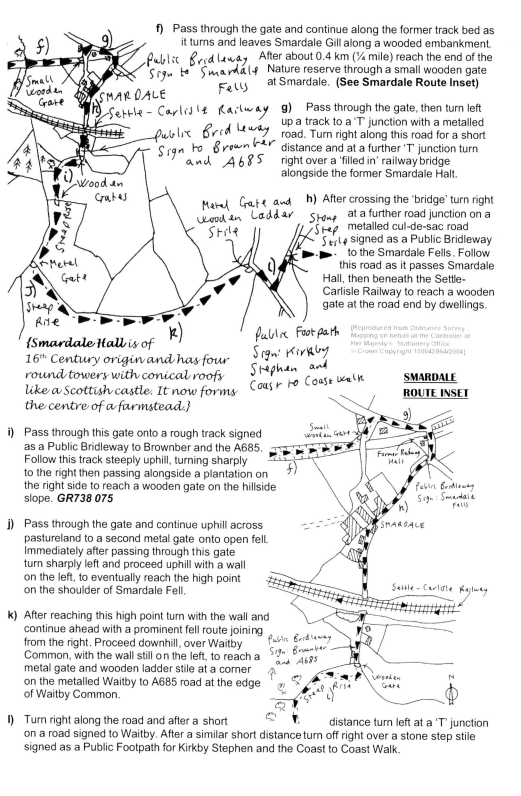

5. Waitby Common to Kirkby Stephen

a) Proceed diagonally left downhill across the field towards a bridge under the Settle-Carlisle Railway rounding the outside corner of a further field before reaching a wooden stile and the bridge.

b) Pass beneath the Railway then veer diagonally to the right across a further field, with ancient settlement remains to the right, to reach a stone step stile by the field corner. **GR756 075**

c) Climb over the stile onto Kirkby Stephen Intake then veer left and downhill and climb over a wooden stile. Continue along the foot of then the right side of a shallow dry valley. Turn to the right upon nearing a further stone wall and cross a small shoulder to reach a combined stone step stile and small wooden gate in the wall ahead.

d) Pass through the gate and proceed downhill on the right side of a pasture, then through a wooden gate onto a track. Pass between the bridge abutments of the former Eden Valley Railway to a metal gate at the entrance to Greenriggs farm complex. **(See Greenriggs Route Inset)**

e) Pass through the gate into the farm yard, turn right and through a second metal gate. Turn left and pass through a third such gate onto the concrete farm access road.

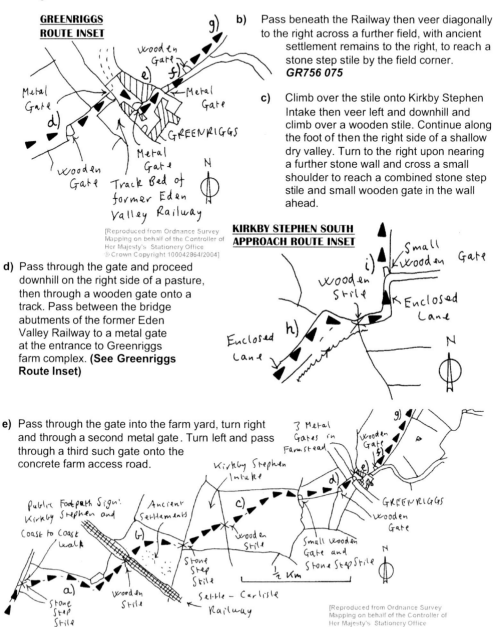

f) Follow this road a short distance to a wooden gate in the left hand wall. Pass through this gate, then continue in the same direction as before, but in the field the other side of the wall.

g) Proceed slightly uphill along the side of the field, at first with a wall on the right, then a fence (and hedge), then thirdly just a broken hedge. Eventually reach a gated stone gap stile at the end of the field.

h) Go through the stile and cross a narrow field to a further stone gap stile. Continue downhill with a wall on the left and stream on the right. Pass through an enclosed stretch of path then turn to the right at a corner to reach a wooden stile at the commencement of an enclosed lane. *GR768083* (See Kirkby Stephen South Approach Route Inset)

i) Follow the enclosed lane a short distance to a sharp right hand corner then turn off through a small wooden gate. Follow the right edge of pastureland to a further small wooden gate by a large tree in the pasture corner.

j) Pass through the gate and after a further short distance along the edge of the pastureland turn off to the right over a wooden stile. Proceed ahead along the right edge of school playing fields. **(See Kirkby Stephen School Route Inset)**

k) Pass open playing fields then fenced all weather pitches. After passing the latter, move across to the right then take an enclosed path in the same direction between boundary fences of a rough car park and farmland. Follow this path to a point level with the gateway of the car park.

l) At the gateway turn sharp left, cross the gateway then follow a further enclosed path between the car park and animal pens. Reach a wooden stile and after climbing over the stile turn right and proceed along a metalled path to reach once again the Kirkby Stephen back road, Faraday Road.

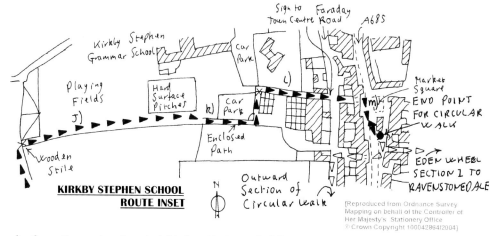

KIRKBY STEPHEN SCHOOL ROUTE INSET

m) Cross the road and go straight ahead between buildings on a path signed to Town Centre. Pass beneath an archway into Market Square then turn right and cross the A685 road at a light controlled crossing to reach the Tourist Information Centre and starting point of the circular walk.

The Countryside Code

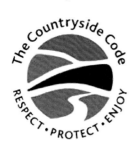

Advice for the public

- Be safe - plan ahead and follow any signs
- Leave gates and property as you find them
- Protect plants and animals, and take your litter home
- Keep dogs under close control
- Consider other people

Countryside Access Charter

Your rights of way are:
- Public footpaths — on foot only. Sometimes waymarked in yellow
- Bridleways — on foot, horseback and pedal cycle. Sometimes waymarked in blue
- Byways (usually old roads), most 'roads used as public paths' and public roads

Use maps, signs and waymarks to check rights of way.
Ordnance Survey Explorer (1:25000 scale) and Landranger (1:50000 scale) maps show mos public rights of way

On rights of way you can:
- take a pram, pushchair or wheelchair if practicable
- take a dog (on a lead or under close control)
- take a short route round an illegal obstruction or remove it sufficiently to get past

You have a right to go for recreation to:
- public parks and open spaces — on foot
- most commons near older towns and cities — on foot and sometimes on horseback
- private land where the owner has a formal agreement with the local authority

In addition you can use the following by local or established custom or consent, but ask for advice if you are unsure:
- many areas of open country, such as moorland, fell and coastal areas, especially those in the care of the National Trust, and some commons
- some woods and forests, especially those owned by the Forestry Commission
- Country Parks and picnic sites
- some private paths and tracks

Eden Wheel South: Circular walks in the series: Length   Time (est.)

		Length	Time (est.)
Walk 1	Kirkby Stephen, Ash Fell & Smardale Gill	21km (13 miles)	6½ hours
Walk 2	Hartley, Nateby Common & Nine Standards Rigg	14km (8.75 miles)	4½ hours
Walk 3	Nateby, Lammerside & Pendragon Castles	14km (8.75 miles)	4½ hours
Walk 4	Wild Boar Fell, Hell Gill & Mallerstang	15km (9.38 miles)	4¾ hours
Walk 5	Ravenstonedale, Crosby Garrett & Scandal Beck	17.5km (11 miles)	5½ hours
Walk 6	Bowderdale, Randygill Top & Weasdale	14km (8.75 miles)	4½ hours
Walk 7	Tebay, Kelleth & the Upper Lune Valley	14km (8.75 miles)	4½ hours
Walk 8	Great Asby, Orton & the Limestone Scars	21km (13 miles)	6½ hours
Walk 9	Roundthwaite, Bretherdale & Borrowdale	15km (9.38 miles)	4¾ hours
Walk 10	Greenholme, Birkbeck Fells and Shap Wells	15km (9.38 miles)	4¾ hours
Walk 11	Swindale, Mosedale & Wet Sleddale	16km (10 miles)	5 hours
Walk 12	Shap, Reagill and Crosby Ravensworth	20km (12.5 miles)	6¼ hours

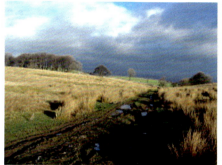
Looking North across fell towards Moor End

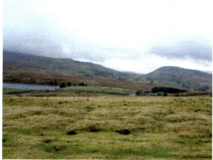
Harter Fell and west slopes of Wild Boar Fell

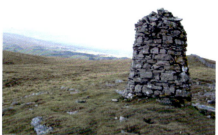
Jack's Cairn, Windy Hill, Ash Fell Edge

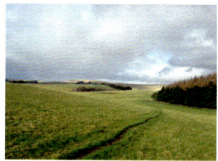
"Ravenstonedale Park"

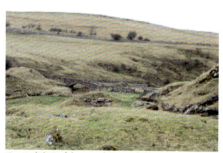
Smardale Bridge and Scandal Beck

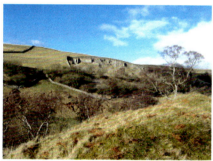
Disused quarries, Smardale Gill

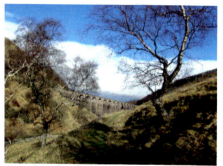
Smardalegill Viaduct

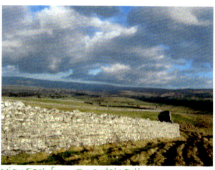
View East from Smardale Fell

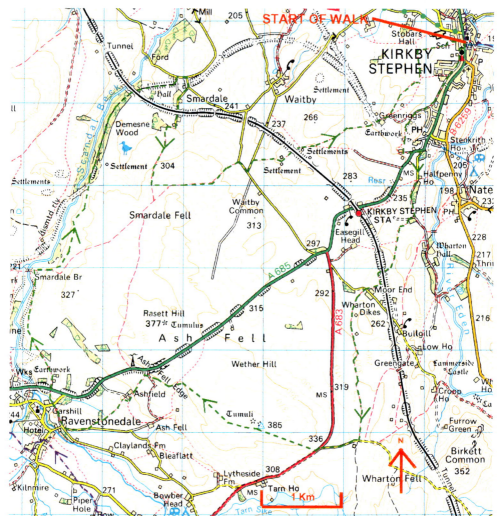

Reproduced from Ordnance Survey based mapping on behalf of the Controller of Her Majesty's Stationery Office © Crown Copyright 100042964/2004

KEY   ---------   Ash Fell and Smardale Gill Circular Walk Route

---------   Eden Wheel Long Distance Walk Route

ISBN 1-905083-00-9

Printed by *cerberus*   Kirkby Stephen, Cumbria